with

Multiple Sclerosis

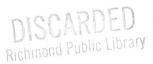

Lisa M. Shulman, MD

Editor-in-Chief, *Neurology Now™* Books Series
Fellow of the American Academy of Neurology
Professor of Neurology
The Eugenia Brin Professor in Parkinson's Disease and Movement Disorders
The Rosalyn Newman Distinguished Scholar in Parkinson's Disease
Director, University of Maryland PD & Movement Disorders Center
University of Maryland School of Medicine
Baltimore, MD

Other Titles in the *Neurology Now™* Books Series

Navigating Life with Parkinson's Disease
Sortirios A. Parashos, MD, PhD; Rose Wichmann, PT; and Todd Melby

Navigating Life with a Brain Tumor
Lynne P. Taylor, MD, FAAN; Alyx B. Porter Umphrey, MD; and Diane Richard

Navigating the Complexities of Stroke
Louis R. Caplan, MD, FAAN

Navigating Life with Multiple Sclerosis

Kathleen Costello, MS, ANP-BC, MSCN

Associate Vice-President, National Multiple Sclerosis Society
Nurse Practitioner, The Johns Hopkins Multiple Sclerosis Center
Baltimore, MD

Ben W. Thrower, MD

Medical Director
Andrew C. Carlos Multiple Sclerosis Institute at Shepherd Center
Atlanta, GA

Barbara S. Giesser, MD

Clinical Director, UCLA Multiple Sclerosis Program
David Geffen UCLA School of Medicine
Los Angeles, CA

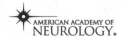

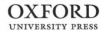

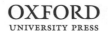

OXFORD
UNIVERSITY PRESS

Oxford University Press is a department of the University of
Oxford. It furthers the University's objective of excellence in research,
scholarship, and education by publishing worldwide.

Oxford   New York

Auckland   Cape Town   Dar es Salaam   Hong Kong   Karachi
Kuala Lumpur   Madrid   Melbourne   Mexico City   Nairobi
New Delhi   Shanghai   Taipei   Toronto

With offices in

Argentina   Austria   Brazil   Chile   Czech Republic   France   Greece
Guatemala   Hungary   Italy   Japan   Poland   Portugal   Singapore
South Korea   Switzerland   Thailand   Turkey   Ukraine   Vietnam

Oxford is a registered trademark of Oxford University Press
in the UK and certain other countries.

Published in the United States of America by
Oxford University Press
198 Madison Avenue, New York, NY 10016

© American Academy of Neurology 2015

Library of Congress Cataloging-in-Publication Data
Costello, Kathleen, author.
Navigating life with multiple sclerosis / Kathleen Costello, Ben W. Thrower,
Barbara S. Giesser.
p. ; cm. — (Neurology now books series)
ISBN 978–0–19–938173–9
I. Thrower, Ben W., author.   II. Giesser, Barbara S., author.   III. Title.
IV. Series: Neurology now books.
[DNLM: 1. Multiple Sclerosis—diagnosis—Popular Works.   2. Multiple
Sclerosis—therapy—Popular Works. WL 360]
RC377
616.8′34—dc23
2014036627

The science of medicine is a rapidly changing field. As new research and clinical experience broaden
our knowledge, changes in treatment and drug therapy occur. The author and publisher of this
work have checked with sources believed to be reliable in their efforts to provide information that
is accurate and complete and in accordance with the standards accepted at the time of publication.
However, in light of the possibility of human error or changes in the practice of medicine, neither
the author, nor the publisher, nor any other party who has been involved in the preparation or
publication of this work warrants that the information contained herein is in every respect accurate
or complete. Readers are encouraged to confirm the information contained herein with other
reliable sources, and are strongly advised to check the product information sheet provided by the
pharmaceutical company for each drug they plan to administer.

3 5 7 9 8 6 4 2
Printed in the United States of America
on acid-free paper

CONTENTS

ABOUT THE AAN'S *NEUROLOGY NOW*™ BOOKS SERIES

Here is a question for you:

If you know more about your neurologic condition, will you do better than if you know less?

Well, not simply optimism but hard data show that individuals who are more knowledgeable about their medical conditions *do have better outcomes*. So learning about your neurologic condition plays an important role in doing the very best you can. The main purpose of both the *Neurology Now*™ Books series and *Neurology Now* magazine from American Academy of Neurology (AAN) and American Brain Foundation (ABF) is to focus on the needs of people with neurologic disorders. Our goal is to view neurologic issues through the eyes of people with neurologic problems, in order to understand and respond to their practical day-to-day needs.

So, you are probably saying, *"Of course, knowledge is a good thing, but how can it change the course of my disease?"* Well, health care is really a two-way street. After you have had a stroke, you need to find a knowledgeable and trusted neurologist; however, no physician can overcome the obstacle of working with inaccurate or incomplete information. Your physician is working to navigate the clues you provide in your own words combined with the clues from their neurologic examination, in order to arrive at an accurate diagnosis

and respond to your individual needs. Many types of important clu
exist, such as your description of your symptoms or your ability to
identify how your neurologic condition affects your daily activities. Poor patient–physician communication inevitably results in
less-than-ideal outcomes. This problem is well described by the old
adage, "garbage in, garbage out." The better you pin down and communicate your main problem(s), the more likely you are to walk out
of your doctor's office with the plan that is right for you. Your neurologist is the expert in your disorder, but you and your family are
the experts in "you." Physician decision making is not a "one shoe
fits all" enterprise, yet when accurate, individualized information is
lacking, that's what it becomes.

Whether you are startled by hearing a new diagnosis or you
come to this knowledge gradually, learning that you have a neurologic problem is jarring. Many neurologic disorders are chronic;
you aren't simply adjusting to something new—you will need to
deal with this disorder for the foreseeable future. In certain ways,
life has changed. Now, there are two crucial "next steps": the first
is finding good neurologic care for your problem, and the second
is successfully adjusting to living with your condition. This second
step depends on attaining knowledge of your condition, learning
new skills to manage the condition, and finding the flexibility and
resourcefulness to restore your quality of life. When successful, you
regain your equilibrium and restore a sense of confidence and control that is the cornerstone of well-being.

When healthy adjustment does not occur following a new diagnosis, a sense of feeling out of control and overwhelmed often per-
sists, and no doctor's prescription will adequately respond to this
problem. Individuals who acquire good self-management skills are
often able to recognize and understand new symptoms and take
appropriate action. Conversely, those who are lacking in confidence
may respond to the same symptom with a growing sense of anxiety and urgency. In the first case, "watchful waiting" or a call to the
physician may result in resolution of the problem. In the second

case, the uncertainty and anxiety often lead to multiple physician consultations, unnecessary new prescriptions, social withdrawal, or unwarranted hospitalization. Outcomes can be dramatically different depending on knowledge and preparedness.

Managing a neurologic disorder is new territory, and you should not be surprised that you need to be equipped with new information and a new skill set to effectively manage your condition. You will need to learn new words that describe both your symptoms and their treatment to communicate effectively with the members of your medical team. You will also need to learn how to gather accurate information about your condition when you need it and to avoid misinformation. Although all of your physicians document your progress in their medical records, keeping a personal journal about your neurologic condition will help you summarize and track all your medical information in one place. When you bring this journal with you as you go to see your physician, you will be able to provide more accurate information about your history and previous treatment. Your active and informed involvement in your care and decision making results in a better quality of care and better outcomes.

Your neurologic condition is likely to pose new challenges in daily activities, including interactions in your family, your workplace, and your social and recreational activities. How can you best manage your symptoms or your medication dosing schedule in the context of your normal activities? When should you disclose your diagnosis to others? *Neurology Now* Books provide you with the background you need, including the experiences of others who have faced similar problems, to guide you through this unfamiliar terrain. Our goal is to give you the resources you need to "take your doctor with you" when you confront these new challenges. We are committed to answering the questions and concerns of individuals living with neurologic disorders and their families in each volume of the *Neurology Now* Books series. We want you to be as prepared and confident as possible to participate with your doctors in your medical care. Much care is taken to develop each book with you in mind. We include the most up-to-date, informative, and useful answers to the questions that most concern you—whether you find yourself in the unexpected role of patient or caregiver. Real-life experiences of patients and families are found throughout the text to illustrate important points. And feedback based on correspondence from *Neurology Now* magazine readers informs topics for new books and is integral to our quality improvement. These features are found in all books in the *Neurology Now* Books series so that you can expect the same quality and patient-centered approach in every volume.

I hope that you have arrived at a new understanding of why "knowledge is empowering" when it comes to your medical care and that *Neurology Now* Books will serve as an important foundation for the new skills you need to be effective in managing a neurologic condition.

Lisa M. Shulman, MD
Editor-in-Chief, *Neurology Now*™ Books Series
Fellow of the American Academy of Neurology
Professor of Neurology
The Eugenia Brin Professor in Parkinson's Disease
and Movement Disorders
The Rosalyn Newman Distinguished Scholar
in Parkinson's Disease
Director, University of Maryland PD &
Movement Disorders Center
University of Maryland School of Medicine

PREFACE: NAVIGATING LIFE WITH MS

The dictionary defines :"navigate" as "steering a course through, finding a way, and directing safely and carefully". Living with Multiple Sclerosis is indeed a journey. Initially the terrain is unfamiliar and the way ahead is not clear. There may be many unexpected events, some frank scares, and times and places where one can feel hopelessly lost. The purpose of this book is indeed to be a "navigator' for your journey with MS. Our hope is that it will help provide a road map as you follow your path.

We've attempted to define the landscape by describing what MS is and how it affects the nervous system. Our signposts are things you should know about symptoms and medications, and ways you can partner with your health care professionals to optimize your health. We present strategies to manage MS, MS symptoms and promote over all well-being.

As with any journey, there are those who can partner with your along the way. This can include your family, friends and your health care providers. Over time, empowered knowledge, and in partnership with your team, you will find that the unfamiliar becomes less intimidating and you will begin to navigate on your own. But, as the saying goes, " A journey of 1000 miles starts with the first step". We hope that this book will be part of your first steps in navigating a full, healthy and fulfilling life with MS.

Navigating Life with
Multiple Sclerosis

Chapter 1

What Is Multiple Sclerosis?

In this chapter, you'll learn:

- **What the term "multiple sclerosis" means**
- **Who is likely to get multiple sclerosis**
- **What causes multiple sclerosis**
- **What are the different courses that multiple sclerosis can take**

If you are reading this book, it is likely that either you or a family member or loved one has been diagnosed with **multiple sclerosis**, also referred to as MS. Perhaps you have lived with MS for years, continuing to search for new information about your condition and ways to manage it. Or the words "multiple sclerosis" may be very new—at least as a term that affects your day-to-day life.

No matter where you are on your journey with MS, this book is intended to guide you through the questions you may have and the decisions you may need to make and to lead you to resources that will help you along the way.

If you're like many people with MS, it may have taken a long time for you to get this diagnosis. Because the symptoms of the disease can come and go unpredictably, people often live with them for years—and may receive several different diagnoses—before their condition is finally identified.

So What Is Multiple Sclerosis, Anyway?

Multiple sclerosis is a chronic disease that affects the body's central nervous system (CNS), which includes the brain, spinal cord, and optic nerves. Actually, it is an **autoimmune disease**, which means that the body's immune system is mistakenly attacking and damaging healthy tissues. This nerve damage can produce many different symptoms, including fatigue, numbness, weakness, vision change, and loss of balance, among others. The time course of the disease is unpredictable and occurring in separate episodes; overall disease severity often varies from one individual to the next.

Multiple sclerosis was first formally described in 1868 by the French neurologist Jean-Martin Charcot, a clinical and scientific pioneer known as the founder of modern neurology. Integrating his clinical and anatomic observations with earlier reports from other nineteenth-century neurologists, he named the condition *la sclérose en plaques disséminées* (disseminated cerebrospinal sclerosis). "Sclerosis" refers to a hardening of the tissues—in this case, the lesions or scars found in the white matter of the CNS. These areas of sclerosis are also referred to as "plaques."

Who Gets Multiple Sclerosis?

According to the National Multiple Sclerosis Society, approximately 400,000 people in the United States today have been diagnosed with MS. About 10,000 new cases are diagnosed each year—that's about 200 people every week. Worldwide, the disease affects an estimated 2.1 million people. Most people with MS are diagnosed when they are between 15 and 50 years old, with the majority of those cases occurring between ages 20 and 40. Susceptibility to MS appears to be influenced by multiple factors, including gender, race, genes, environment, and possibly some lifestyle choices.

Gender

Multiple sclerosis is a sexist disease; it affects almost three times as many women as men. For reasons that are not yet entirely clear, most autoimmune diseases are more common in women. Recent research suggests that this may be a result of profound effects on immune function by both sex hormones and sex chromosomes.

Race

Multiple sclerosis is much more common in whites than persons of other races. For example, it is very rare among Inuit populations. It is also more common among whites who have northern European or Scandinavian ancestry. This underscores the role of genetics in contributing to MS susceptibility.

Genes

In the general population, the risk of developing MS is about 0.1%, or 1 out of 1,000 people. A person who has a first-degree relative with MS, such as a parent or sibling, has about a 4% chance of developing MS. Should both parents have MS, each of their children will have 30% to 35% chance of developing MS. It is important to note that, while some genetic association exists, there is no conclusive evidence to date that the disease can be inherited from a parent through gene transmission. But several studies have identified certain genes—that are part of regions on **chromosomes** called the **major histocompatibility complex (MHC)**, which controls the development and function of many immune components—that are more common in people with MS than in the general population.

Environment

For reasons that are not completely understood, the farther one lives from the equator, the higher one's chances are of getting MS. The place where a person lives before age 15 appears to particularly influence susceptibility. For instance, someone who lives in Florida until he or she is 15 years old and then moves to Montana keeps a lower "Florida risk" of MS for the rest of his or her life. On the other hand, someone who lives in Montana until age 15 and then moves to Florida carries the higher relative "Montana risk." To summarize, the person who moves after age 15—whether nearer to or farther from the equator—retains the relative risk associated with the place where he or she spent time growing up until age 15. This geographic difference in risk may be due to a higher risk of viral infections or lower vitamin D levels as one lives further from the equator. So a composite "typical" person with MS might be a 28-year-old white woman who was born and grew up in Minnesota and whose ancestors were Swedish.

Lifestyle

Recent research findings suggest that smoking increases the risk for developing MS, including secondhand smoke and possibly even prenatal exposure. There are also studies that have reported that girls who are obese as children or adolescents have a higher risk of developing MS. While these observations are not yet definitive, they underscore the importance of maintaining a healthy lifestyle and may hold important clues to the underlying mechanisms that produce nerve damage in MS.

What Causes Multiple Sclerosis?

In multiple sclerosis, the body's immune system attacks the CNS and destroys a substance called **myelin**, which forms a protective sheath around the nerve fibers known as axons—the primary transmission lines for the electrical signals within the nervous system. The axons, as well as **oligodendrocytes** (the cells that make myelin) can also be damaged or destroyed in MS.

Scar tissues, or **plaques**, form where the myelin has been damaged. The damage to myelin and axons disrupts or stops altogether the signals transmitted from one nerve cell to the next. Think of it as a downed power line—when that power line is damaged or cut, it can't transmit the signal telling your refrigerator or telephone to turn on. Similarly, if enough nerve cells are damaged in your CNS, signals that tell you to move your arm or maintain your balance can be interrupted.

The exact cause of MS remains unknown. However, many researchers think that a combination of genetic and environmental factors is responsible for the autoimmune process that causes the damage to the CNS, resulting in the symptoms that are characteristic of this disease.

For example, because people who live in more northern climates appear to be more susceptible to MS, scientists are studying the idea that low vitamin D levels may be linked to the disease. Naturally produced vitamin D, which is created by exposure to sunlight, is thought to have a beneficial effect on the immune system and thus may protect against autoimmune diseases like MS. Given that people who move from a darker, more northern climate to a sunnier one at a young age acquire the relative risk for MS found in their new, adopted climate, it might make sense that something about vitamin D levels during a certain key period of childhood and young adulthood plays a role in developing MS. Many different studies have now reported that low sunlight exposure in early childhood, and thus lower Vitamin D levels during this time, appears to correlate with an increased risk of developing MS later in life.

Viruses are also thought to have a possible link to MS. (This does not mean that MS is contagious!) There are two ways in which a virus might cause the nerve damage that is seen in MS.

One is that the virus might attack the nervous system directly. But there is an indirect way in which a virus can cause damage. When a virus enters the body, the immune system becomes activated in order to fight its invasion. In MS, some of the immune system cells mistake certain cells and tissues of the CNS as invaders and respond by attacking them. One trigger for this mistaken immune response might be if a component of the CNS mistakenly viewed the immune cells as part of a virus, the so-called by-stander immune response. Today, researchers are studying more than a dozen viruses to determine whether any of them might trigger the onset of MS in someone who already carries a genetic susceptibility. Although **epidemiologic studies**—studies of whole populations—suggest that exposure to some type of infection might play a role in MS, no single virus has yet been definitively linked to the disease.

What Are the Types and Stages of Multiple Sclerosis?

Multiple sclerosis does not have one predictable disease course. The nature of multiple sclerosis and the patterns it takes vary from person to person. Traditionally, doctors have described four different courses of disease in MS, based on how the disease begins and how the symptoms of the disease occur over time. The four types were relapsing-remitting, progressive-relapsing, primary progressive, and secondary progressive MS. In 2013, the National MS Society (NMSS) recommended changing these categories so that the progressive-relapsing category was dropped. Three types are used in the new classification scheme; clinically isolated syndrome, relapsing-remitting, and progressive MS. Progressive MS is divided into primary and secondary. The NMSS suggests further classification based upon whether the disease is active (relapses and/or new lesions on MRI) and whether the MS is still progressing or not. Let's look at these types of MS. We will talk about clinically isolated syndromes in Chapter 3.

Relapsing-Remitting Multiple Sclerosis

Between 85% and 90% of individuals newly diagnosed with MS are said to have what is called the **relapsing-remitting** course of the disease. A relapse occurs when an individual develops neurologic symptoms that last a minimum of 24 hours and cannot be explained by any other cause, such as an infection. During these relapses, neurologic function is impaired—for example, a person may have great difficulty walking without tripping or find it difficult to see clearly out of one eye. Relapses generally last as long as several weeks and then begin to resolve or disappear. Symptoms may go away completely or partially. After a relapse subsides, long periods of time—even years—may pass in which no new symptoms typical of a relapse occur. These periods are called remissions. Old symptoms may still be present during these remissions.

Susan was diagnosed with MS after experiencing an episode of **optic neuritis** (inflammation of the optic nerve causing vision impairment in one eye) that was followed 6 months later by numbness in both her legs.

The optic neuritis began when Susan awoke one morning and noticed that the vision in her left eye was blurry, as though her contact lens was dirty. And when she looked around, she had an achy sensation behind that eye. She saw an ophthalmologist and was found to have visual acuity or sharpness of vision of 20/200 in the left eye as well as impaired color vision—both findings being characteristic of optic neuritis.

(Continued)

(Continued)

After about six weeks, the optic neuritis went away, and Susan recovered her vision almost completely. Because optic neuritis can be a common first symptom of MS, Susan's ophthalmologist referred her to a **neurologist**, who ordered an **MRI** scan of her brain. The MRI showed evidence of plaques in the brain that were compatible with MS. But with only one symptom, the diagnosis of MS could not be made (see Chapter 3 for further details).

Six months later, Susan woke up with a numb left foot. Over the next 2 days, this numbness spread to both legs and up to her waist. She again went to see her neurologist, who believed that with the two episodes (optic neuritis and numb legs), Susan had a definite diagnosis of MS. These symptoms persisted for 4 weeks and then subsided, leaving a slight numbness in her left large toe. She has not experienced any additional symptoms since that time.

Susan's optic neuritis and episode of numbness are each examples of relapses. The periods of time in between the relapses and following the last relapse are called remissions (or recovery). Recovery may or may not be 100%, although recovery is often better early in the disease. When recovery is less than 100%, it is considered incomplete, and the remaining symptoms are termed **residual symptoms**.

Secondary-Progressive Multiple Sclerosis

Over time, many people with relapsing-remitting MS tend to see the number of relapses and remissions they experience diminish. The initial phase of ups and downs is followed by a course, called **secondary-progressive MS**, in which the disease worsens over time and may include **periodic plateaus** (periods when the disease is stable), occasional relapses, and minor remissions.

Research in people who were untreated showed that in half of those with relapsing-remitting MS transition to secondary-progressive MS within about 10 to 15 years of the first symptom and that about 90% do so within 20 years. To most of us, the word "progression," when linked to a disease, sounds ominous; and in MS may imply that life in a wheelchair lies ahead. However, that is not always how things end up. In fact, even though many people with relapsing-remitting MS will move on to a secondary-progressive disease course, far fewer will ultimately need a wheelchair.

Jane was diagnosed with MS at the age of 31. During the next 10 years she experienced four relapses, including a band of numbness around the waist, weakness of the right arm and leg, optic neuritis of the left eye, and clumsiness of the left arm and hand. Each of these relapses lasted several weeks and then remitted over several more weeks. Jane had incomplete recovery from two of the relapses and continued to experience mild weakness of the right arm and leg and occasional numbness around her waist.

Following her last relapse, Jane noticed over the next 2 years that her walking endurance declined, and she slowly developed more weakness in her right upper and lower extremities, to the point that she now sometimes trips over her right foot when walking. She also finds that she can no longer hold objects with just her right hand. As time has passed, she has begun to need to use a cane when walking farther than two blocks.

(Continued)

> *(Continued)*
> Jane's MS can now be described as secondary-progressive. She had clear relapses early in the disease, but after 10 years, she began to have a decline in function even without experiencing another obvious relapse.

Primary-Progressive Multiple Sclerosis

As mentioned, initial diagnoses in about 85% to 90% of cases are identified as relapsing-remitting MS. Approximately 10% of the remaining cases are categorized as **primary-progressive MS**, a course marked by a slow decline in neurologic function from the start, with no sharply identifiable relapses or remissions. The condition may plateau or even temporarily improve at times, but the symptoms generally do not diminish. Individuals on this course of the disease often experience difficulties with their ability to walk over time. Unlike the other types of MS, primary-progressive multiple sclerosis appears to affect men just as often as women. The initial onset of primary-progressive MS also differs somewhat from other forms of the disease; it tends to be diagnosed more often after age 40, about 10 years later than other forms of MS. Also, primary-progressive MS almost always affects the spinal cord, which tends to produce problems with mobility as well as bladder, bowel, and sexual dysfunction. Someone with primary-progressive MS may need the assistance of a cane or crutch when walking sooner after being diagnosed than someone who is diagnosed with the relapsing-remitting form.

> Steve, who is in his mid-40s, began to experience problems during his daily 5-mile run. His legs became unnaturally stiff and tired, and he needed to shorten his run to 3 miles. He
> *(Continued)*

(Continued)

also noticed that his legs tingled when he jogged. The symptoms seemed to go away about 4 hours after he finished a run, only to return the next time he went out. Over a period of 18 months, the tingling and stiffness increased. But he did not seek medical help until his wife, after noticing that his manner of walking, or **gait**, seemed to be growing unsteady, persuaded him to see his primary care physician. The doctor watched Steve walk and then tested his strength and reflexes. She asked if he had ever experienced double vision, vision loss, muscle weakness, or other neurologically related problems. He was unable to recall having had any such difficulties. The doctor referred Steve to a neurologist, who performed an MRI that revealed the kinds of lesions in both the brain and spinal cord that MS produces.

Seeing the lesions that are typical of MS, the neurologist also performed a **lumbar puncture** and numerous blood tests to rule out other diseases. After evaluating the various test data, the neurologist told Steve that he had primary-progressive MS, based on the fact that there had been no definitive relapse-remission phase and that Steve's neurologic symptoms had worsened relatively slowly from the time he had first seen clues of a problem during his daily run.

What Type of Multiple Sclerosis Do I Have?

The course of the disease is not always simple to define. This is particularly true when trying to distinguish between relapsing-remitting and secondary-progressive MS, as incomplete recovery from relapses often occurs and can be difficult to distinguish from progression. Progression of symptoms may be subtle or quite slow. Often the course of the disease becomes clearer over years. Over a year or more, progression can usually be identified that would characterize secondary-progressive MS. Primary-progressive MS may also require time to establish the course is without relapses.

How Multiple Sclerosis Symptoms Change Over Time

People newly diagnosed with MS summon up mental pictures of the disease that are formed by their knowledge and past impressions. The image of a family member, friend, acquaintance, or public figure who has had MS will likely come to mind first. More often than not, these initial images prompt fear. The first question people who have been diagnosed most commonly ask neurologists is, "When will I be in a wheelchair?" People worry whether they will be able to continue working, raising their families, and participating in all the other activities that make up their lives.

While it is true that MS is a chronic disease—meaning that, once diagnosed, it will remain with you for the rest of your life—it is neither a death sentence nor a one-way ticket to a wheelchair. Most people with MS develop coping strategies for dealing with relapses and with changes that occur over time and lead very productive, satisfying lives—having children, pursuing careers, and enjoying sports and hobbies.

How Do I Learn Whether I Have Multiple Sclerosis?

If you're reading this book, it's likely that you've already been given a diagnosis of MS or have a loved one who has received such a diagnosis. But if you're still wondering, it's time to get answers.

The diagnosis of MS can sometimes be difficult to make. There is no single test that can diagnose MS, and symptoms that ultimately are part of a diagnosis of MS may be unclear at first and may even look like a different disease process. The basic rules for establishing a diagnosis of MS are two different episodes of neurological symptoms that occur at different times and are from different areas of the central nervous system- and must not be due to another cause. The history of symptoms is then combined with any findings from the neurologist's examination of the patient, abnormalities found on an MRI of the brain and spinal cord, blood tests to exclude other diseases, and sometimes other tests such as a lumbar puncture (spinal tap, used to obtain spinal fluid for testing).

When Should I See My Doctor?

If you are experiencing a change in your vision, sensation, strength, coordination, or walking you need to make a medical appointment to learn what might be causing the symptoms.

Although it may be frightening to think of being diagnosed with a serious, chronic neurologic condition like MS, knowledge is power. The more you know, the more you can do to help take control of your condition. Also, the earlier MS is diagnosed, the sooner specific treatment can be initiated that can help slow down or stop nerve damage. You'll learn more about diagnosing MS in Chapter 3.

Summary

Multiple sclerosis is a complex disease of the CNS that is caused by abnormal function of the immune system. Much has been learned about MS since it was first described in 1868. However, important questions such as what causes MS have not been completely answered. Although MS is a chronic condition that will be with the patient for the rest of his or her life, it is not generally fatal nor does it mean that a person will inevitably end up in a wheelchair. Due to new and effective treatments that can slow nerve damage and help to manage symptoms, most people with MS lead full and productive lives.

Chapter 2

How Multiple Sclerosis Affects the Nerves

In this chapter, you'll learn:

- **How the nervous system is organized**
- **How the immune system and inflammation are involved in the development of multiple sclerosis**
- **How multiple sclerosis damages the central nervous system**

How the Nervous System is Organized

Multiple sclerosis (MS) is a disease of the **central nervous system (CNS)**, so to understand MS it is essential to first understand how the nervous system works.

The nervous system is composed of two parts: the CNS and the **peripheral nervous system (PNS)**. The CNS comprises the brain, the spinal cord, and the optic nerves (Figure 2–1). The brain is the body's command center. It interprets and processes messages that arrive through the spinal cord and special sensory organs such as the eyes and ears and responds to this information. Incoming information is sensory; outgoing information is motor. The incoming and outgoing information is transmitted to and from the PNS via pathways in the spinal cord (Figure 2–2).

The PNS has two components, the **somatosensory nervous system** and the **autonomic nervous system.** The somatosensory nervous system is composed in part of twelve pairs of **cranial nerves**

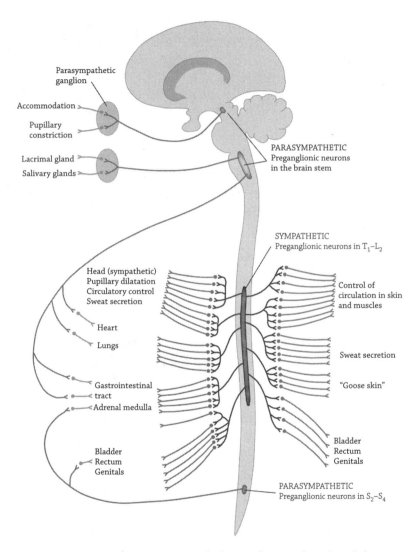

FIGURE 2–1 The CNS comprises the brain, the spinal cord, and the optic nerve.

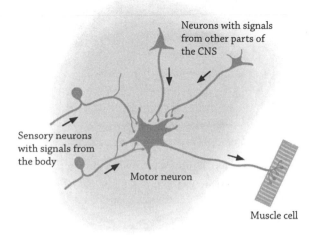

Neurons with signals from other parts of the CNS

Sensory neurons with signals from the body

Motor neuron

Muscle cell

FIGURE 2-2 Convergence of neural connections.

that control sensation and movement of the head and neck as well as eye movement, taste, smell, and vision. Nerves coming out from the spinal cord make up the remainder of the somatosensory system. They relay sensory information from the body to the brain and send motor messages from the brain to the muscles to control movement. The highly complex operations of these interrelated systems are responsible for receiving and interpreting stimuli and transmitting **nerve impulses** (or signals) throughout the body.

For example, if you touch a hot stove, a nerve impulse travels from your fingers via the peripheral nerves and through the spinal cord to your brain, telling it that the stimulus is painful, and your brain instantly sends a returning signal to your hand, jerking it away from the burner.

The autonomic or automatic nervous system controls the heart, breathing, digestion, and waste elimination, transmitting messages to the various organs that regulate the workings of our bodies. Multiple sclerosis less frequently affects the autonomic nervous system.

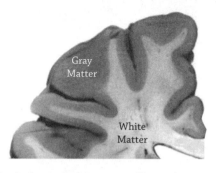

FIGURE 2-3 In the brain, a thin outer ribbon of gray matter surrounds a large inner mass of white matter.

The two main types of tissue found in the CNS are **gray matter** and **white matter**. In the brain, a thin outer ribbon of gray matter surrounds a large inner mass of white matter (Figure 2–3). The gray matter is composed of **nerve cells** that direct all bodily functions. The white matter is made up of thousands of wirelike extensions of the nerve cells—called nerve fibers (or **axons**)—that send electrical and chemical messages from one part of the brain to another. One of the important functions of white matter is to facilitate communication between different parts of the brain. Nerve fibers in the brain and spinal cord are wrapped in layers of myelin, a fatty substance that both protects the fibers and accelerates nerve-impulse transmission (Figure 2–4). More of the myelin is found in white matter, and this is the main target that is attacked in MS. The myelin in the PNS is just different enough from the myelin in the CNS so that nerves in the PNS are not attacked in MS. So essentially, MS is primarily a disease of CNS white matter, although, recently, advanced imaging techniques have identified gray matter damage from MS. Unfortunately, when an axon loses its myelin, it becomes vulnerable, and the axon can be damaged too. Also, it has been discovered that axons can be injured in MS even when they have not lost their myelin, by mechanisms that have yet to be fully understood.

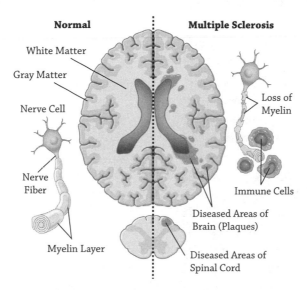

FIGURE 2-4 Nerve fibers in the brain and spinal cord are wrapped in layers of myelin, a fatty substance that both protects the fibers and accelerates nerve-impulse transmission.

The Immune System and Multiple Sclerosis

The job of a normally functioning immune system is to protect the body (self) from "nonself" invaders, such as bacteria, viruses, and other foreign substances. In a healthy individual, immune cells have very limited ability to get into the CNS. Most researchers agree that in MS, the **immune system** mistakes myelin and other substances in the CNS as foreign and produces an autoimmune ("self" immune) response that damages and destroys myelin and axons. This is called an autoimmune ("self" immune) response. Exactly how does this happen?

The major "players" in the autoimmune response in MS are types of white blood cells called T cells and B cells. T cells, so called because they mature in the thymus gland, can become helper T cells, which promote the immune response; regulatory T cells, which help diminish the immune response; or cytotoxic T cells, which directly attack other cells or foreign substances. Persons with MS have been shown to have higher numbers of helper T cells and lower numbers of regulatory T cells, especially during an MS attack or exacerbation.

Immune system cells respond to the presence of an antigen (a substance perceived as non-self) by producing a highly coordinated response that includes inflammation. In MS it is believed that T cells respond to self- antigens in the CNS, such as the proteins in myelin. When a T cell recognizes an antigen, it becomes activated and multiplies. An army of T cells is then formed to "search and destroy" the identified antigen. In MS the army is able to cross into the CNS from the blood vessels and when they encounter a CNS antigen that they recognize, an immune attack begins with the release of inflammatory substances from the T cells. Other types of immune cells are signaled to assist in the attack and ultimately myelin and axons are damaged and destroyed. Since the antigen is in the CNS, the activated T cell has to have the ability to get into the CNS, something a nonactivated T cell normally cannot do. A network of very small blood vessels called the **blood-brain barrier** does exactly what that name implies in healthy individuals, that is, it keeps unwanted entities (such as immune cells) out of the CNS. In people with MS, the immune cells can get through the blood-brain barrier and into the CNS to attack myelin and axons (Figure 2–5). Some of the disease-modifying therapies (discussed in Chapter 5) work by preventing immune cells from getting into the CNS. The precise mechanisms whereby the T cells become sensitized to the CNS antigen, and exactly which CNS antigen(s) are involved, are still not fully understood and are targets of much research activity.

B cells, produced in the bone marrow, primarily contribute to immune function by producing antibodies (immune proteins), which are also involved in damage to myelin and axons. B cells have also been shown to secrete other nonantibody substances that are toxic to myelin-forming cells and may have other ways in which they participate in the autoimmune response that are not

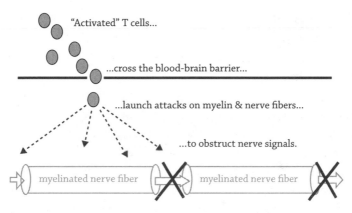

FIGURE 2–5 Immune steps leading to neurologic deficits.

yet fully understood. Several large ongoing clinical trials are look-ing at specific anti-B-cell agents to determine their efficacy as disease-modifying therapies.

In the normal immune system, regulatory mechanisms keep the body's own cells and tissues from being mistaken for foreign invaders and thus prevent autoimmune activity (activity directed against the body itself) and diseases. However, when the immune system malfunctions and the regulatory mechanisms fail, auto-immune activity is the result. Autoimmune activity can be directed at a variety of different cells, tissues, and body systems, and researchers are still trying to discover why certain areas are targeted. Many diseases other than MS are considered autoim-mune, such as rheumatoid arthritis, lupus, Crohn's disease, and psoriasis.

How Does the Immune System Cause Nerve Damage?

Most researchers think that MS-related damage to the CNS is caused, at least in part, by **inflammation**. When the immune system recognizes an injury or a foreign invader, or **antigen**, it triggers a series of events in the body that result in inflammation, which directs immune cells and immune proteins to the site of the antigen or injury. Some of these immune cells actually surround and digest the antigen and any damaged tissue around it. Inflammation is a sign that the body is working to rid itself of the invader. Often, this is a good thing—if inflammation never occurred, cuts and wounds would never heal and tissue damage would continue. But chronic inflammation that is directed against the wrong target—like in MS—can ultimately damage and destroy normal tissue. Normally the CNS has mechanisms, particularly specialized blood vessels that prevent most immune cells and immune proteins from entering. But in MS, the immune cells are able to sneak into the CNS, where they produces inflammation and nerve damage that leads to neurologic symptoms.

The damaged myelin is replaced by areas of scar tissue (plaques), which build up over the nerve fibers (axons) and impede the axons' ability to transmit electrical impulses. Consequently, nerve impulse transmission along a damaged axon may be slowed, misinterpreted, or stopped altogether. Think of a frayed telephone wire. If there is some damage to the insulation around the wire, the signals may be slowed in reaching the receiver or they may be distorted ("static"). If enough of the insulation and the wire is damaged or the wire is cut, the signal transmission will stop altogether.

When enough disruption and blockage of these nerve signals has occurred, MS symptoms occur. The type of symptom is determined by which area of the nervous system is affected. For example, if the **optic nerve** is harmed, a loss of vision may occur. If damage has occurred in the spinal cord, the ability to walk may be compromised.

Because inflammation is one of the main mechanisms by which nerves are damaged in MS, anti-inflammatory medications are often used as treatments. Steroids have powerful anti-inflammatory properties, and are often given during an acute MS attack, when much inflammation occurs. Steroids help to accelerate recovery from the acute attack, but only have a short-term effect. The disease-modifying therapies (see Chapter 5) also have anti-inflammatory effects and work over the long term.

Not all areas of the CNS affected by MS produce noticeable symptoms, in part because there is redundancy in much of the brain (meaning there is more brain tissue than we actually use). Even in areas that are damaged as a result of MS, there is the ability for the body to repair some of the damage. When an axon is demyelinated, its ability to transmit information becomes disrupted. In response to this, there is some ability to reorganize the message pathway. In addition, some remyelination of an axon can take place, especially if enough of the myelin-forming cells, or oligodendrocytes, are still present and functioning.

The brain can also reorganize and activate additional areas of the brain to assist an area that has undergone some damage—a process known as "plasticity." These repair and reorganization mechanisms, while very helpful, are not quite as effective as the original areas of nerve function and are more susceptible to future damage. Brain plasticity is also limited by additional inflammation and damage that may occur with the MS disease process.

Much knowledge has been gained over the past few decades about the way in which MS causes nerve damage. As a result, researchers have already discovered agents that limit ongoing inflammation and damage, such as the currently available disease-modifying agents discussed in Chapter 5. Now, researchers are looking to determine what triggers the immune attack on the nerves and are doing research to develop mechanisms to protect nerves and even repair the damage that has occurred. For example, stem cell therapy may one day be able to replace or repair nerve damage in persons with MS. Several agents are in development that may stimulate or promote remyelination. Other ways are being studied to expand the capacity for plasticity so that new nerve pathways can take over the functions of damaged ones. Some research even suggests that simple everyday activities such as exercise and certain lifestyle choices may be useful in helping to promote nerve protection and plasticity (see Chapter 6).

Summary

Multiple sclerosis is so named because it may damage multiple parts of the CNS. Often the areas of nerve damage do not produce any symptoms, but can be seen on MRI pictures. Much research is ongoing to discover ways to protect nerves from damage and also to expand the natural repair capabilities already present in the CNS.

Chapter 3

How Multiple Sclerosis Is Diagnosed

In this chapter, you'll learn:

- **What the "rules" are for making a diagnosis of multiple sclerosis**
- **Why your physician has recommended certain tests, examinations, and procedures**

You may have already been diagnosed with multiple sclerosis (MS), or you may currently be involved in the diagnostic process. In either case, it may seem confusing and uncertain. As there is no single diagnostic test for MS, zeroing in on the diagnosis is challenging. Despite the many medical advances in the specialty of MS care and research that have occurred since the 1990s, arriving at the diagnosis continues to cause much frustration. Because some symptoms that ultimately turn out to be MS can be vague at first and are also seen in other conditions, it may take months and sometimes years before MS can be confirmed. Making a timely diagnosis is important so that treatment can be initiated early in the disease process, and in the absence of a specific diagnostic test, medical experts in MS and MRI (magnetic resonance imaging) have developed guidelines for establishing a diagnosis. The basic "rules" are that there must be objective evidence of damage to the central nervous system (CNS; that is, brain, spinal cord, and optic nerve) in more than one place, and occurring at more than one point in time. (Remember, it's called *multiple* sclerosis for a reason!) Also, other diseases that might produce the same findings have to be eliminated as possible causes. This information is gathered from various sources, beginning with an individual's history of symptoms and a neurologic examination. If the history and the examination suggest MS, then additional tests, such as an MRI of the brain and spinal cord, a lumbar puncture (done to test the spinal fluid), and an **evoked potential study,** which tests the nerve pathways from the vision, hearing, or sensation centers to the brain, may be done to help support or exclude the suspected diagnosis. A number of blood tests are conducted to exclude other conditions that may mimic MS, such as some infections or other diseases that cause inflammation.

Clinically Isolated Syndrome

Sara is a healthy 35-year-old woman. She is married with two small children and holds a full-time job. One morning as she is toweling off after her shower, she notices numbness in her legs. Over the next two days, the numbness spreads to include her hips. By the fourth day, the numbness reaches to her waist. She also feels a sensation of heaviness in her legs, but the sensation does not interfere with her ability to walk or other usual activities. Several times over the next 10 days, she considers making a doctor's appointment but never quite gets around to it. After about 3 weeks the symptoms gradually disappear.

"I'll bet my legs were acting up because of that new aerobics class I started," she thinks. "But they're fine now."

Ultimately, Sara may experience additional symptoms that are more clearly attributable to a problem in the CNS. But at this point in time, she has only experienced a single episode referable to the CNS (the tingling in the legs).

When someone has a first neurologic attack, such as Sara's, that is consistent with CNS inflammation, it is considered a **clinically isolated syndrome** or CIS. Most, but not all people who experience

CIS will later develop more symptoms and more evidence of CNS inflammation and thus may be diagnosed with MS. A CIS is a clinical symptom or symptoms that arise from an abnormality in the brain or spinal cord. A CIS can involve one symptom, such as visual loss in one eye, or can involve more that one symptom such as weakness and visual symptoms. The key is that the symptoms occur at the same time. When one symptom is involved it is considered monofocal. When more than one symptom is involved it is considered multifocal. While this presentation can be highly suggestive of MS, the symptoms must be separated in space *and* time. A CIS does not fulfill the "separation in time" criterion necessary for the diagnosis of MS.

Abnormalities consistent with the inflammation and demyelination seen in MS that emerge on brain MRI and/or in the spinal fluid can be highly predictive for MS. Research has shown that starting treatment in a person who has had a CIS and whose brain MRI shows abnormalities will extend the time before the next attack occurs. Identification of a CIS is an early opportunity to institute disease-modifying therapies—the medications that reduce the immune system attacks on the nerves. All of the self-injected medications, namely, beta interferons and glatiramer acetate (as well as one of the newer oral medications [teriflunimide], Chapter 5) have been tested in well-designed clinical trials in people who have experienced a CIS (Table 3–1). These studies have demonstrated that intervention at the time of a CIS can delay the next clinical event and reduce the development of new CNS inflammatory changes and damage.

Sara, like many people with early relapsing-remitting MS, may now go months or years before experiencing any other symptoms. Even if she had seen a doctor during that first week, MS might not have been suspected as the first—or even the second—possible source of her numbness and heavy sensation. Sara may experience other symptoms, such as fatigue, which is the most common symptom of MS. But because fatigue can be such a vague symptom and is easy to attribute to other causes, it may not prompt a visit to the doctor. Even if it does, fatigue alone may not lead to an investigation for MS.

TABLE 3-1 Emerging Therapies

Treatment	Stage of Development	How It Works
Anti-LINGO[1]	Phase 1	May help repair myelin
Daclizumab[2]	Phase 2, 3 (Relapsing-remitting multiple sclerosis)	Inhibits T cells in the immune system
Ocrelizumab[3]	Phase 2, 3 (Relapsing-remitting multiple sclerosis, primary-progressive multiple sclerosis)	Inhibits B cells in the immune system
BAF312 (siponimod)[4]	Phase 1, 2 (Relapsing-remitting multiple sclerosis) Phase 3 (Secondary-progressive multiple sclerosis)	Prevents some lymphocytes from causing inflammation, similar to fingolimod
ONO–4641[5]	Phase 2	Prevents some lymphocytes from causing inflammation, similar to fingolimod
Ponesimod[6]	Phase 2	Prevents some lymphocytes from causing inflammation, similar to fingolimod
XP23829[7,8]	Phase 1	May work as an antioxidant, similar to dimethyl fumaric acid

When symptoms occur that seem to be due to a CNS process, such as blurred vision in one eye, double vision, or numbness (like that experienced by Sara), MS may be on the list of diagnostic possibilities. However, other conditions may be on that list as well. Some of the conditions that may show symptoms similar to MS, particularly early on, include other autoimmune disorders, such as rheumatoid arthritis and lupus; vascular conditions, such as abnormal blood vessels in the brain or migraine headaches; metabolic disorders, such as vitamin B_{12} deficiency; infections, such as Lyme disease; and even CNS tumors. These other possibilities must be excluded before the diagnosis of MS can be confirmed.

Since MS is an unpredictable disease affecting the CNS (the brain, spinal cord, and optic nerve) and there is no specific diagnostic test, how is it diagnosed? Remember, to make a diagnosis there must be objective evidence of the occurrence of at least two neurologic events separated in space and time. Let's look at how the clinical story, or presentation, and the neurologic examination and tests such as MRI can be used to confirm or rule out a diagnosis of MS.

First, the symptoms of relapsing-remitting MS can come and go; this is the "time" part. For example, a person who had a brief episode of leg numbness a year ago may, this year, have an episode of vision loss in one eye. In addition, MS affects different parts of the CNS; this is the "space" part. For example, leg numbness may be due to a problem in the spinal cord, whereas the vision loss may be linked to a problem in the optic nerve.

Another simple but important fact is that an MS diagnosis cannot be made on the basis of symptoms alone. There must be objective evidence to explain the symptoms, such as an abnormal neurologic examination and evidence on an MRI scan of the CNS that is consistent with MS. Other tests may be done that can also help in making the diagnosis, such as a lumbar puncture or an evoked potential study. These tests will be discussed in greater detail later in this chapter.

About 6 months after the episode of numbness in her legs, Sara has the onset of blurred vision and pain in in one eye. When this does not go away after a few days, she goes to her ophthalmologist, who looks in her eyes and sees evidence of inflammation of the optic nerve in one eye (optic neuritis). Because of this, Sara is referred to a neurologist, who orders an MRI. When the MRI of the brain shows lesions typical of MS, this, coupled with the history of two different episodes of neurologic symptoms, enables the neurologist to confirm a diagnosis of MS.

The Initial Diagnosis of Multiple Sclerosis

While early diagnosis of MS is important so that appropriate treatment can be initiated, it is also vital that the correct diagnosis be made. Careful exclusion of conditions that can mimic MS must be done prior to making the diagnosis. This is accomplished through blood tests, MRI, and sometimes by analysis of spinal fluid following a lumbar puncture.

If you experience neurologic symptoms such as visual loss or blurring in one eye, double vision, numbness or tingling in an arm or leg, weakness, or difficulty with coordination (or other symptoms that you are unsure of) that lasts greater than 24 hours, it is important to seek medical attention. While symptoms such as these could be an indication of many different disorders, MS is one of the possible diagnoses.

History of Symptoms

When you are evaluated by your doctor for possible MS or any possible diagnosis, the first thing any physician will do is take a detailed history of symptoms. The doctor will ask many questions about the current symptoms, which may include the following:

- When did the symptoms begin?
- Have you ever had them before?
- Do the symptoms interfere with your usual activities?
- What have you done to alleviate the symptoms?
- Have your interventions helped?
- Have you had any recent infections?
- Have you been diagnosed with any other illnesses recently?

In addition, the doctor will ask whether you have ever had any other symptoms that might be characteristic of a CNS problem and whether any family member has ever had similar symptoms or any other illnesses, especially MS or other autoimmune diseases, like rheumatoid arthritis or lupus. The doctor will ask if you have any allergies and also what medications, vitamins, and any other dietary supplements you take and why. The doctor will also ask about your lifestyle and habits, including diet, exercise, and use of tobacco, alcohol, or other recreational substances.

As noted, even though MS can manifest itself in a wide variety of ways, some common patterns exist. For example, it is much more prevalent among young adults (the age of diagnosis generally ranges from 20 to 50, with the average age of onset in the mid-30s). An 80-year-old man exhibiting new neurologic symptoms is more likely to have something other than MS. Typical MS attacks evolve over several days or more and last days, weeks, or even up to a month or more. A person who sees sparkles of light for 15 minutes and then has a throbbing pain behind the eyes probably has migraine headaches, not MS.

Physical and Neurologic Examination

After collecting the history, the doctor will conduct an examination to evaluate your neurologic function. You will be asked questions to determine how clearly you are thinking. Your vision, hearing, speech, head and neck mobility, arm and leg mobility, strength, coordination, and your ability to walk all will be carefully evaluated. The doctor will tap certain places on the arms and legs to test your reflexes. Typically, the deep tendon reflexes, tested with taps from a rubber hammer to specific areas of the upper and lower extremities, are somewhat overactive in persons with MS. Abnormal reflexes, such as an positive Babinski sign—that is, the upward movement of the big toe and fanning out of the other toes when the underside of the foot is stroked, may appear. The doctor will touch your skin with a pin, to see how well you can sense a sharp sensation, and touch specific bones in the upper and lower extremities with a tuning fork, to see whether you can distinguish vibration.

During the physical exam, the doctor looks for clues that may point either toward or away from a diagnosis of MS. For example, an examination of the eyes may show changes that suggest MS. Using an instrument called an ophthalmoscope your healthcare provider can see the optic disk, located in the back of the eye and the back of your eye, or retina. The optic disk examination can provide valuable information about the optic nerves (the nerves from each eye that carry visual information to the vision center in the brain). Inflammation of the optic nerve from optic neuritis causes swelling of the optic nerve as well as the optic disk. Damage from a prior bout of optic neuritis may cause the optic disk to appear paler than is normal.

Also, a patient may have had previous episodes of neurologic damage that did not produce symptoms but that left behind clues visible on the neurologic examination. For example, the pale optic disc described above might be seen in a patient who never experienced a noticeable episode of vision loss. The physical examination may also yield clues that point away from the diagnosis of MS. Absent or diminished deep tendon reflexes, for instance, along with a loss of sensation on examination, may suggest damage in the peripheral nerves called a peripheral neuropathy. Examination of the skin and the presence of certain rashes may point toward some other autoimmune condition, such as lupus.

Based on the symptom history and exam findings, the doctor may refer you to a neurologist, who will ask similar symptom-related questions and likewise perform a neurologic examination. If these, together, point to a problem in the CNS, the neurologist will likely order an MRI. A brain MRI is the type of scan most often chosen. A spinal cord MRI may also be done.

Neurologic examinations that yield abnormal results may not by themselves be enough to make a diagnosis of MS. Diagnosing MS requires putting all of the diagnostic pieces together like a puzzle.

Thus when the exam findings are combined with the history and other diagnostic tests, they can help build a conclusive case.

Magnetic Resonance Imaging (MRI)

The MRI scan is a particularly sensitive diagnostic tool used in the process of determining a diagnosis of MS. It provides physicians with detailed pictures of the brain and spinal cord. MRI uses a strong magnetic field and radio frequencies to generate images. In addition, gadolinium, a contrast agent (dye), injected into a vein of the arm is used to identify areas of active inflammation in the brain and spinal cord. (Radiation is not used in this procedure.)

A brain MRI takes about 40 minutes and spinal cord MRIs take about 40 to 60 minutes. More time may be needed if the brain and spine scans are being done at the same time. You will be asked to lie very still on a table that slides into the scanner. The scanner is a tube that is open on both ends. The tube is narrow but large enough to hold a person weighing up to 300 pounds. The injection of the gadolinium dye may produce a warm sensation throughout the body. Within 5 minutes, images appear that can help the doctor tell whether the MS is in an active phase, even if there have been no recent symptoms. Areas of nerve damage visible on the MRI are called "lesions" or "plaques." A lesion or plaque, in medical speak, means an area of damage or injury, or the evidence that inflammation and demyelination have occurred. Plaques show up as white spots on certain MRI sequences (Figure 3–1).

Newer MS plaques, generally those that have existed less than 6 weeks and those that are actively inflamed will take up the gadolinium dye and appear bright (Figure 3–2). In about 5% of people who are ultimately diagnosed with MS, their MRIs may initially appear normal. However, the longer a person has MS, the less likely it is that his or her MRI will appear normal. New diagnostic criteria allow the diagnosis of MS to be made, even if a person has only had

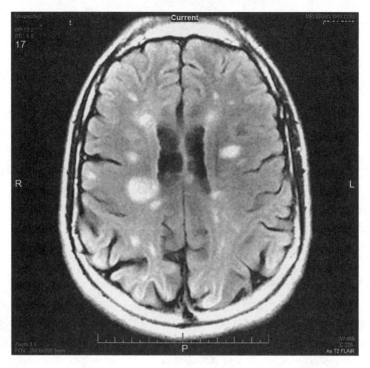

FIGURE 3-1 Plaques show up as white spots on certain MRI sequences.

one attack, if the MRI shows the presence of inflamed and noninflamed lesions at the same time.

Not all white spots that may show up on an MRI are due to MS, however. A long list of conditions, ranging from migraine headaches to stroke, can cause changes that will appear on an MRI. Lesions typical for MS usually appear to be rounded or ovoid (like an oval) in shape. The number of lesions varies among individuals with MS, but multiple lesions are expected. Minor abnormalities of the brain may even be seen on the MRIs of people who have no obvious health problems.

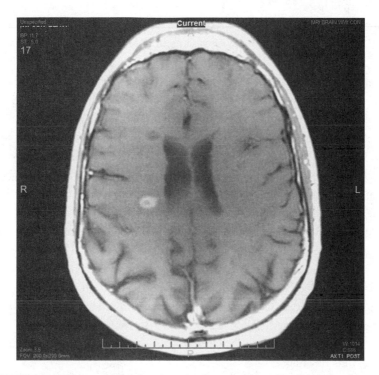

FIGURE 3-2 Newer multiple sclerosis plaques, generally those that have existed less than 6 weeks and those that are actively inflamed, will take up the gadolinium dye and appear bright.

Lumbar Puncture

A lumbar puncture, or spinal tap, is a procedure in which a sample of **cerebrospinal fluid (CSF)** is taken for examination. CSF is a clear fluid that surrounds the brain and spinal cord. In MS, the spinal fluid may show certain abnormalities that can help the neurologist make a correct diagnosis. In many instances, a diagnosis of MS is made without performing a CSF examination; however, a lumbar puncture may be done in order to rule out other conditions that may mimic MS or to provide more evidence of MS when there is insufficient information from other tests and examinations.

For example, in parts of the country such as the northeastern part of the United States, where Lyme disease is found, the lumbar puncture may be used to help distinguish this condition from MS.

The CSF can be studied for evidence of overactivity of the immune system. As discussed in Chapter 2, MS is characterized by an immune attack on myelin in the CNS. This may result in abnormal antibody production in the spinal fluid, which is measured by the presence and rate of production of certain immune proteins in the CSF. CSF that shows any of these abnormalities can strongly suggest MS, although some other autoimmune conditions, like lupus, can also cause the same CSF abnormalities. So a "suspicious" lumbar puncture does not definitively point to MS; instead, it is one important piece of evidence that helps specialists diagnose or rule out the condition. Also, it is important to remember that up to 10% of people who actually have MS can have normal spinal fluid, so if all the other information is consistent with a diagnosis of MS, normal CSF does not negate the diagnosis.

Evoked Potentials

Evoked potentials, also called "evoked responses," are studies of the nerves' response to various stimuli. These can be visual, such as a flashing light; auditory, such as a click or a tone; or sensory, such as an electrical pulse to the arm or leg. Each type of response is detected by recording brain waves that are generated by the brain in response to the stimulus, using electrodes that are pasted to the head. Normally, nerve impulses are transmitted from one point to another in the spinal cord and brain without being impeded. Lesions associated with MS may slow or block that transmission, so a prolonged or absent evoked potential response indicates nerve damage. Evoked potential studies are used to detect evidence of demyelination in specific parts of the CNS that may not show up on the history, examination, or MRI. Therefore, they are very useful for detecting clinically silent lesions; that is, areas of nerve damage that do not produce symptoms or are too small to be seen on an MRI. For example, when Sara went to her doctor with complaints of numbness in her legs, that symptom would have been caused by a spinal cord lesion. Sara had not had any visual symptoms, and the doctor didn't see anything wrong when he looked in her eyes. But when the visual evoked response test was done, it was slowed, indicating that Sara had had an old inflammation of the optic nerve, even though it hadn't produced any symptoms. In this case, the evoked potential provided evidence of a clinically silent lesion that was the second area of nerve damage, thus helping to fulfill the criterion of "separation in space" for making the diagnosis of MS.

Blood Tests

The neurologist will also order a number of blood tests to rule out diagnoses of conditions that can produce symptoms similar to those indicative of MS. Blood is drawn for evidence of Lyme disease and other infections, vitamin deficiencies, other inflammatory diseases such as lupus, and certain metabolic and inherited diseases. Currently there is no blood test that can diagnose MS, although this is an active area of investigation.

Putting the Picture Together

Once all of these examinations have been completed, your neurologist will put all of the evidence together to determine whether or not you should be diagnosed with MS. As mentioned earlier in this chapter, MS clinical and MRI experts have established written guidelines to aid physicians in making this diagnosis. The guidelines have been revised several times as technological advances have improved and provide more help in establishing or excluding an MS diagnosis.

Currently, MS experts use an updated version of guidelines known as the McDonald Criteria, named after their lead author. These criteria give fairly specific rules for using the history, neurologic examination, MRI, CSF examination, and evoked potentials to produce a diagnosis. New criteria allow certain MRI findings to fulfill the requirement for separation in time on a single scan, without having to wait for additional symptom or repeated MRI scans. But the basic principles are the same, and there has to be documentation of damage to the brain, spinal cord, or optic nerve in more than one place and occurring at two different time points, without another disease process being able to account for the findings.

The time it takes to make the diagnosis of MS has been reduced as knowledge about the disease and diagnostic testing has improved. It is important to pursue the diagnosis, because if MS is confirmed, treatment can be initiated. Based on multiple research studies, early treatment of MS is felt to be better in the long run than waiting to start treatment. In MS, much of the inflammation and damage occurs without any outward symptoms. Thus, MS is similar to an iceberg: What we see on the surface are the symptoms of the disease, but the true extent of the disease includes not only the symptoms but also the disease process that lies below the surface. Because this damage will increase over time, it is important to treat the disease as early as possible.

The treatments for MS do not change the symptoms of the disease, but they do reduce new inflammation that will cause additional damage. While they are not cures, the medications for MS are effective treatments and do reduce the number of relapses and new areas of inflammation and they can help prevent worsening over time. Research has indicated that the number of early relapses and early changes seen on MRI are predictive of the level of disability that can occur over time. While these predictors are not always 100% accurate, most MS specialists and researchers agree that early intervention is better than waiting to begin treatment. Given the importance of early diagnosis and treatment of MS, scientists are looking for ways to identify the disease as early as possible. It is important to make the diagnosis of MS as quickly as possible, but also as accurately as possible. An incorrect MS diagnosis may lead to unnecessary treatment of the wrong health issue. Researchers are trying to identify biomarkers (substances or cells in the brain, blood, or spinal fluid that may appear early in the disease and/or MRI findings that are more specific for MS so that the diagnosis can be made as quickly and accurately as possible.

Summary

While no one specific, "sure fire" test exists to diagnose MS, there are well-established guidelines, and most of the time a diagnosis is made in a timely fashion. Accurate diagnosis is important not only to initiate specific treatment for MS but also to establish whether other conditions are present so that their treatment may be started instead. Diagnostic methods continue to improve; for example, MRIs are much more sensitive now than they were a decade ago, and much research is being devoted to finding markers that are more sensitive and specific for MS to make the diagnostic process easier and faster for both patients and physicians.

Chapter 4

Managing Multiple Sclerosis Symptoms

In this chapter, you'll learn:

- **What the most common symptoms of multiple sclerosis are**
- **How to use medication, rehabilitation, and other strategies to treat symptoms and optimize function and safety**

If you have recently been diagnosed with multiple sclerosis (MS), you probably have many questions. For instance, you may be wondering, What symptoms can I expect? How can the symptoms be treated? Will I get worse? Will I need a wheelchair? Will I continue to be able to work?

In this chapter, we will discuss all of these questions and more, helping you learn about living with MS. We'll also talk about strategies for alleviating and coping with common MS symptoms, including medications, rehabilitation strategies, and cognitive retraining.

People who have MS generally find that the symptoms affect them in several primary areas: mobility, sensation, vision, cognition (thinking functions such as memory and processing speed), mood, and genitourinary (GU)—that is, bladder, bowel, and sexual—function. This chapter discusses the symptoms that can produce impaired function in these areas, except for mood, which will be discussed in detail in Chapter 6.

How Multiple Sclerosis Affects Mobility

Many of the symptoms of MS are invisible to others. Often, you cannot just look at someone with MS and immediately detect fatigue, pain, or cognitive challenges. On the other hand, when someone uses a cane, walker, wheelchair, or scooter, it is clear that the limbs have been affected by the disease. So it's not surprising that among the first questions are those around mobility issues.

It is important to remember that in many cases, an MS diagnosis is not a one-way ticket to impaired mobility. Although there really is no way of accurately predicting any one person's course of MS symptoms, the reassuring fact is that 20 years after diagnosis, about two-thirds of people with MS will *not* need a wheelchair.

Nonetheless, most people with MS do experience some kind of change in their mobility—either temporarily during a relapse or more permanently as the disease progresses. Most people take walking and moving their arms for granted, not realizing how many neurological functions are involved in these routine motions. Strength, sensation, coordination, balance, proprioception, (the ability to detect changes in position), and muscle tone all play a role in the ability to move and walk, and MS may affect one or more of them. It is worth taking a brief look at how each of these functions should operate, how MS can affect a given function, and what can be done to deal with those effects.

Strength

At the simplest level, muscles move when they receive signals from the brain that tell them to. Multiple sclerosis interferes with signal transmission. The damage is done both by demyelination—the destruction of **myelin**, the fatty insulating substance that protects nerve fibers (axons) in the brain and spinal cord and helps them transmit signals—and damage to the underlying axons themselves. When myelin is missing or damaged, the signals transmitted throughout the central nervous system (CNS) are disrupted or halted and the brain becomes unable to send and to receive messages.

These "signal interruptions" can cause problems with both intentional and reflexive leg and arm movements. Weakness can result when nerve signals have trouble getting from the brain to the muscle. A person with MS may find that strength varies widely, even over the course of a single day: In the morning, picking up a heavy object may be possible, but in the afternoon, after a long walk or an hour sitting out in the sun, lifting the arms or getting out of a chair is difficult. This is because, although demyelinated axons can still send signals, overexertion or exposure to excessive heat may shut them down temporarily. When the strength of a person with MS is tested in a cool, relaxed examination room, it may seem fine. However, if the same person is tested right after a vigorous walk, the results might well reveal a weakness that was not obvious before. A drug that has been shown to improve walking by improving the electrical conduction in demyelinated nerves is called Ampyra (dalfampridine).

Two muscle groups that play a major part in walking and are especially susceptible to weakening because of MS are the hip flexors and the ankle dorsiflexors. The hip flexor muscles help bring the knee toward the abdomen, while the ankle dorsiflexors bring the toes and feet off the ground. Ankle dorsiflexor weakness results in **footdrop**. If a person with footdrop has strong hip flexors, he or she is able to raise the knee high enough to avoid dragging the toes. The hip flexors in some people with MS are too weak to enable them to do this; they compensate by swinging the weak leg out, or hiking the hip up on one side, in order to keep their toes from dragging. Both hip flexor weakness and foot dorsiflexor weakness can increase the chances of falling. Working with a rehabilitation specialist of physical therapist is an important part of maintaining strength and balance, and assistive devices can help with footdrop. These and related concerns are discussed in the section "Addressing Mobility Symptoms."

Bob has had primary-progressive MS for the past 12 years and is now 53 years old. An avid runner, he found that he tended to stumble during longer runs. Over the years, his runs have become shorter because of this tendency to drag his left foot. He begins his runs lifting his legs and feet normally, but after about half a mile, he begins to drag the foot and finds the leg feels very stiff. This worsens until he feels he must stop or risk falling.

His neurologist refers Bob to a physical therapist to evaluate his walking. The physical therapist notices that the toes of Bob's left shoe are more scuffed than those on his right. A left footdrop is diagnosed. The physical therapist recommends an assistive device called an ankle foot orthotic to help lift Bob's foot and improve his walking (Figure 4–1). In addition, Bob is shown various exercises to strengthen the leg. While some muscles are not getting the correct signal from the CNS, strengthening exercises can help to maintain function in less-affected muscles to permit safer ambulation.

Balance and Coordination

Demyelination and the resultant formation of scar tissue in the CNS can also produce three symptoms involving muscle movement and coordination: ataxia, tremors, and dysmetria.

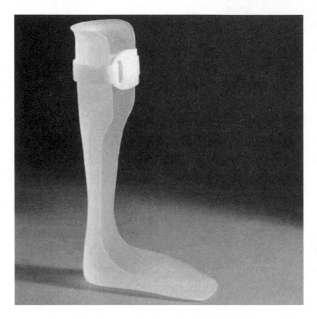

FIGURE 4-1 An ankle-foot orthotic to help lift the foot and improve walking.

Ataxia is disturbance of balance and coordination. It can occur in the limbs, the trunk, or with walking. For example, a person with walking or gait ataxia will appear unsteady and may stumble from side to side. **Tremors** are involuntary rhythmic movements of a given body part, usually an arm or leg, although head tremors may occur as well. **Dysmetria** is the undershooting and overshooting of the intended movement toward a target—for example, you may reach out to shake someone's hand and grab his or her elbow instead. Clearly, all three symptoms can affect mobility. For example, someone whose strength is otherwise normal but who has ataxia or dysmetria (or both) may find walking and other activities difficult because of impaired balance and incoordination.

Danielle was diagnosed with MS 8 years ago and is now 31 years old. She has normal strength in her extremities but has difficulty walking, as she has very poor balance. She stumbles frequently and drifts from side to side. She has fallen several times. After a particularly bad fall, Danielle's husband convinces her to see her doctor. Her doctor believes Danielle may need to walk with an assistive device, such as a walker or cane, but Danielle is opposed to using anything to help her walk and feels as though this would mean she is "giving in" to her MS. Her doctor recommends physical therapy. The physical therapist helps Danielle understand the advantages of using an assistive device, explaining that Danielle is far less likely to fall and would be able to walk without stumbling.

Unfortunately at this time there are no very effective medication treatments for tremors, ataxia, or dysmetria. Sometimes drugs such as diazepam (Valium), clonazepam, and lorazepam may help somewhat with these symptoms, but they can produce sedation and lead to tolerance or dependence. Other drugs that may lessen tremor include propranolol and primidone. For persons who have tremors and dysmetria in their arms, an evaluation by an occupational therapist (OT) can often be very helpful. The OT can recommend strategies and assistive devices that improve upper extremity function and the ability to complete activities such as eating, dressing, and grooming. A physical therapist can provide exercises to improve balance and may use strategies such as a weighted belt to help compensate for ataxia.

Proprioception: A Sense of Self and the Space Around Us

When we purposely move our arms or legs, the brain sends a signal down the spinal cord to the muscles and joints, telling them what parts of the body to move, how fast, and in what direction. In response, other parts of the CNS help guide that movement by providing information about how the body is moving and ensuring that our movements are smooth, controlled, and coordinated. Equally important, the muscles and joints send signals back to the brain telling it where the body part that is to be moved is already positioned. This latter information is called **proprioception** or "position sense."

Are you standing up? Sitting down? Lying down? Bending over? Are your arms over your head? Is the ceiling above you or below you? The sense that tells you all these things is proprioception, and its normal function is essential to coordinated movements, balance, and walking.

Multiple sclerosis can cause significant changes in proprioception, even in people with normal strength, which in turn can have a big impact on the ability to stand, walk, or perform basic activities of daily living. Humans are top-heavy animals: Whenever we stand, we are in a state of nearly falling. As we tilt one way or the other, our changes in position are relayed to the brain, which sends out nerve signals that enable us to take corrective action. All this happens continuously and without our being aware of it.

Multiple sclerosis–related nerve damage that disrupts the transmission of proprioceptive signals to the brain may make a person tilt so far that a fall is inevitable. People with impaired proprioception due to MS are often thought by unknowing observers to have had too much to drink; this is **sensory ataxia**. They use walls, furniture, or the person next to them to keep steady. When the brain isn't receiving the proprioceptive signals it needs for proper balance, visual information becomes more important. Walking in the dark, not looking straight ahead while walking, or standing with your eyes closed (such as when you wash your hair in the shower) all increase your risk of falling when proprioception is poor.

Muscle Tone

Mobility also depends on normal muscle tone, which can be abnormal in persons with MS. One of the primary tasks of your muscles is to either flex a given body part or extend it. Normally, these opposing actions are kept in balance, except when we are consciously moving an arm or leg. **Muscle tone** refers to how loose or stiff the muscles are. Normally, there is a balance between muscles that bend or flex a body part and muscles that straighten or extend a body part. A sudden tightening of muscles, such as in a leg or around the torso, is referred to as a **spasm. Spasticity** is a chronic state of excessive muscle tone (too much tension in the muscles), which is very common in MS—up to 75% of people with MS experience spasticity. Often in MS, spasticity or increased tone is present when the limb is extended away from the body—this is known as increased extensor tone. The degree of spasticity can vary: A leg may suddenly become locked and refuse to bend, or a limb can simply feel stiff and difficult but not impossible to move. Spasticity tends to persist over time, while spasms are briefer spells in which the person is unable to temporarily overcome a flexion or extension posture of an arm or a leg. Spasms, while usually brief, can be painful and recurrent. They often are more frequent during the night and are then known as nocturnal spasms.

Jane was diagnosed with MS 10 years ago and is now 44 years old. Jane experiences spasms in her legs at night, particularly after a busy day that includes extensive walking. She finds that her legs cramp behind her knees during the night, interrupting her sleep. Sometimes, her toes even curl and she needs to pry them into a normal position with her hands. Jane reports these symptoms to her doctor, who prescribes the medication tizanidine to be taken at bedtime to relieve some of the muscle tightness. In addition, he recommends that she see a physical therapist who can teach her stretching exercises.

Certain medications that can be helpful in treating spasticity are discussed in the following section, "Addressing Mobility Symptoms."

Raymond was diagnosed with MS 20 years ago and is now 47 years old. He has some weakness in the legs but is able to walk with a cane or walker. His legs feel stiff or tight, especially after prolonged sitting or when he first gets up in the morning. In addition, he has waves of intense spasms in his legs, mostly at night. His neurologist recommends a trial of baclofen. The medication does help with both the spasticity and spasms, however Raymond notes that his legs feel too loose or rubbery since he started the new medication. An adjustment to a lower dose results in good control of the muscle tightness with no weakness.

Excessive extensor tone in the legs can be both a good and a bad thing. If MS has resulted in leg weakness, you may use that extensor leg tone to help stand and walk; however, too much leg stiffness may result in difficulty getting your feet to move when walking. Another way spasticity can impair walking is by causing scissoring—the feet moving to cross over each other instead of moving ahead parallel to each other.

Addressing Mobility Symptoms

Multiple sclerosis can affect mobility by causing muscle weakness, faulty coordination, disrupted proprioception, and spasticity. All these symptoms can be addressed, and potentially alleviated, through physical therapy, assistive devices, and to some extent with medications.

Working with a Physical Therapist

A referral to a knowledgeable rehabilitation specialist or physical therapist who is familiar with MS is important—even when an individual has no mobility or walking problems—so that the most appropriate exercises and training can be prescribed. A physical therapist can recommend exercises that can be useful for maintaining strength and flexibility before mobility problems occur. If problems with increased spasticity or mobility do occur, the individual already has an established physical therapy provider who can modify the treatment plan to meet the new challenges. When working with a physical therapist, people who have MS who do have mobility problems can, first of all, identify the factors that are affecting their ability to get around and then develop a routine of exercises specifically aimed at improving strength, flexibility, muscle control, and balance.

There is no one right exercise for all people with MS. The physical therapist will help tailor a program that best fits the needs of an individual. An individual exercise routine will contain some mixture of stretching, strengthening, and cardiovascular exercises as well as specific strategies directed at compensating for specific deficits. For example, the physical therapist may instruct a patient to move his legs in a certain way while walking to compensate for weakness or loss of balance.

There are some important principles to remember when someone with MS exercises. While most of us want to be in better shape, the "no pain, no gain" adage will not work in MS. Exercising to the point of exhaustion in MS could produce excessive fatigue, such that the individual may not be able to participate in normal daily activities. Vigorous exercises can also produce excessive heat that can cause weakness and fatigue for many living with MS. Thus developing an exercise plan with a rehabilitation specialist who is knowledgeable about MS will likely produce the best exercise program for each individual.

Assistive Technologies

A common goal when a person with MS is evaluated by a rehabilitation specialist is to walk better. Sometimes in order to accomplish this goal, some people will need assistive devices to help their mobility. While many people will not need an assistive device, numerous devices are available for those who do, including ankle-foot orthotics (for foot drop), wireless stimulators for upper and/or lower leg weakness, straight canes, forearm crutches, rollators, scooters, and both manual or electric wheelchairs.

For some people with MS—like Danielle, introduced earlier in this chapter—the idea of using an assistive device feels like "giving up" or "letting MS win." While this is understandable, assistive devices can also mean triumph over the limitations of MS. Without an assistive device, some people with MS may find themselves shut out of many enjoyable activities, such as sporting events, family gatherings, and shopping. If a walker or cane allows someone to attend their child's soccer game or their 20th class reunion, that's not a loss—it's a win. Think of an assistive device as the right tool for your "job"—getting where you want to go and doing what you need to do, safe from falls and injury.

The use of an assistive device is a personal decision—one that therapists, doctors, and nurses may encourage, but one that is often avoided by the person living with MS. But using an assistive device to help with walking may allow you to be much more physically active. The device may help to normalize walking, reduce discomfort, and reduce fatigue. Improved endurance may allow for greater participation in the activities once avoided.

Those trying to decide whether to begin using an assistive device should be sure to seek information and guidance from their doctors and physical therapists. A rehabilitation specialist who is familiar with gait disturbances seen in MS should make an assessment for an assistive device. As MS functional abilities can vary from day to day, sometimes several types of assistive devices are necessary. Even a device as simple as a cane should be obtained with a prescription, so that the correct type of cane—with the correct height, handle, and base—can be used.

Wheeled devices require an evaluation by a rehabilitation specialist such as a physical therapist so that the correct seat, arm or leg rests, cushions, and other accessories and chair weight can be determined. The rehabilitation specialist will work collaboratively with the referring neurologist so that a prescription specific to the individual's needs can be written. Motorized devices are very expensive, and while most insurers will cover the device, they will not cover multiple motorized devices. Thus determining the correct device is very important. Issues to consider include cost, portability, and the ability to maneuver the motorized device inside the home. Devices should never be ordered online without the input and careful evaluation of a rehabilitation specialist familiar with motorized devices.

Leg weakness particularly footdrop—is very common in MS. Recent technological advances have been made that can be quite useful for some individuals with MS. An ankle-foot orthotic has been the usual device used for footdrop. The ankle-foot orthotic is an L-shaped plastic or lightweight carbon device that fits under the foot and up the back of the weak leg to prevent the foot from "dropping" forward. Thus during the gait cycle, the toe is prevented from dropping, and tripping is prevented.

Two wireless electronic devices have been developed that may also be helpful. The WalkAide and BioNess L300 devices use wireless technology to electrically stimulate the peroneal nerve in the leg, which activates the muscles that lift the foot. With these devices, a sensor in the shoe detects when the foot comes off the floor just prior to its coming forward in the gait cycle. The sensor sends a wireless signal to a device worn around the upper calf, just below the knee. The signal causes the device to electrically stimulate the peroneal nerve as it exits the muscle in the upper calf. When this nerve is stimulated, it stimulates the muscle that lifts the toe upward. While these high-tech electrical devices are a wonderful development and may be preferable to standard ankle-foot orthotics, they are not appropriate for everyone. They are costly, and insurance coverage is not guaranteed in all cases. Appeal letters from doctors and therapists are often necessary to request insurance coverage for the WalkAide or BioNess L300, and many times the cost must be covered by the individual. It is important to work with an experienced rehabilitation specialist to determine whether the wireless devices are appropriate for the individual gait abnormality and then plan the appropriate appeal strategy.

As mentioned previously, hip flexion weakness can also interfere with the ability to walk. A hip flexion assist device (HFAD) may help compensate for this. The HFAD is a belt worn around the waist and has an elastic band that extends down from the belt and is attached to the top of a person's shoe on the affected leg. The tension on the elastic band helps bring the hip up to assist in walking (Figure 4–2).

Medications

Certain medications can also help improve mobility for people with spasticity. Antispasticity drugs such as baclofen or tizanidine (Zanaflex) are taken to lessen spasticity. Baclofen can be taken orally, but large doses may result in drowsiness. Another form of baclofen is delivered into the fluid space around the spinal cord by means of a surgically implanted pump. This can be very helpful for people who cannot tolerate or are not helped enough by the baclofen taken by mouth. When baclofen is given by pump, its positive effects are achieved with much smaller doses and, frequently, are accompanied by fewer side effects than the oral form of the drug.

Tizanidine, another medication for increased spasticity, which is only given by mouth, can also cause drowsiness and at higher doses may result in a drop in blood pressure. Diazepam, clonazepam, and lorazepam are sometimes used for nocturnal spasms, as they cause significant drowsiness and also last through the night in contrast to shorter-acting medications such as baclofen or tizanidine.

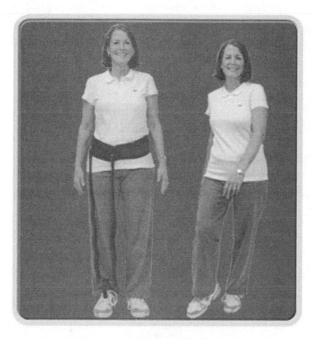

FIGURE 4-2 A hip flexion assist device (HFAD) is a belt worn around the waist that has an elastic band that extends down from the belt and is attached to the top of a person's shoe on the affected leg. The tension on the elastic band helps bring the hip up to assist in walking.
Image used with the kind permission of BTM Rehabilitation, Inc.

Summary

If you are anxious about your walking ability or other mobility issues that could occur due to MS, you are not alone. Multiple sclerosis is unpredictable and highly individualized, and with these characteristics nearly everyone with MS worries about potential future mobility problems, especially when first diagnosed. It's important to remember that motor problems do not happen to everyone with MS and that, when they do occur, many options exist for managing them in a way that can allow you to do the things that you want to do.

When MS affects walking, it is necessary to ascertain whether muscle weakness, faulty coordination, disrupted proprioception, deconditioning, or spasticity—either singly or in combination—is the chief problem. Physical therapy, assistive devices, and medications such as those mentioned above, can all play a role in improving and maintaining mobility.

How Multiple Sclerosis Affects Sensation

In addition to issues with sensation that can affect mobility, people with multiple sclerosis may experience a variety of other sensation disturbances. These alterations may include numbness, **paresthesias** (tingling or prickling), and **dysesthesias** (painful sensations). There used to be a common misconception that MS did not produce pain; regrettably, this is not true; a variety of pain syndromes can result from MS.

As you have already learned, MS alters the way electrical signals are transmitted to and from the body and the CNS because of demyelination and nerve damage. This nerve damage not only disrupts or blocks transmission of electrical signals but can also produce crosstalk between nerves, or a kind of "static," When this happens, sensory abnormalities and decreases in normal sensory function are the result.

These symptoms are not limited to the blunting of normal sensations (in the form of numbness, for instance) but frequently include new sensations, as well. Extra sensations such as tingling or "pins and needles" are called paresthesias. These extra feelings may be just a curious nuisance for some. When extra sensations cause discomfort, they are called dysesthesias. Paresthesias and dysesthesias can take various forms, such as the feeling that a bug is crawling on one's skin, the sense that a hair is tickling the skin, the feeling that the skin is sunburned, or the feeling that electrical shocks are occurring. They can also be manifested as hypersensitivity to touch, or even as allodynia—which is when a normally nonpainful sensation, such as a touch or caress, is painful. A very common dysesthesia is for a person to feel as though he or she is wearing a tight belt or girdle around the chest or abdomen, which is often called the "MS hug." Like many MS-related symptoms, paresthesia and dysesthesia are not unique to MS and can often be seen in other medical conditions.

Diane has had MS for 4 years and is now 31 years old. When she was diagnosed, she was experiencing a tingling sensation in her left foot and leg up to the hip. Since that time, she has had a mild tingling sensation in the toes of her left foot. It is not really painful; rather, she describes it as annoying. Some days it is worse than others. Sometimes when she is very tired or has been up on her feet much of the day, she notices more tingling in the toes in the evening. Once, about 2 years after her diagnosis, she felt discomfort in the toes and at the top of her foot. For a short period, wearing shoes with laces was very uncomfortable and produced a painful electrical sensation in her foot (dysesthesia). This lasted about 2 weeks and then went away, but she now continues to have a constant mild tingling in the toes.

Dysesthesia and paresthesia can be treated with a variety of medications, most of which are categorized either as antidepressants or as anticonvulsants. The way some of these drugs are designed to work against depression and seizures makes them useful for pain management, as well. These medications may lessen any discomfort associated with paresthesia or dysesthesia, but they do not actually restore normal sensation.

Table 4–1 lists of some of the more commonly used medications for uncomfortable sensory symptoms and their possible side effects. These are not complete lists of side effects. The risks and benefits of any medication should be discussed with your neurologist.

If a small area of skin is affected by uncomfortable sensory changes, an over-the-counter topical ointment containing capsaicin

TABLE 4–1 Medications Used for Dysesthesia

Medication	Side Effects
Antidepressants	
Amitriptyline (Elavil)	Dry mouth, drowsiness, blurred vision, constipation, urinary retention, weight gain
Venlafaxine (Effexor)	Nausea, headache, drowsiness, dizziness, loss of appetite, nervousness, weight gain, sexual dysfunction
Duloxetine (Cymbalta)	Nausea, headaches, drowsiness, dry mouth, dizziness, weight gain, sexual dysfunction
Nortriptyline (Pamelor)	Dry mouth, drowsiness, constipation, urinary retention
Anticonvulsants	
Gabapentin (Neurontin)	Dizziness, drowsiness, coordination problems, swelling in the feet/legs, weight gain
Tiagabine hydrochloride (Gabitril)	Dizziness, weakness, tremor, drowsiness
Pregabalin (Lyrica)	Dizziness, drowsiness, problems with coordination, weight gain
Carbamazepine (Tegretol/Carbatrol)	Dizziness, drowsiness, unsteadiness, nausea, skin rash, abnormal blood counts
Oxcarbazepine (Trileptal)	Headaches, drowsiness, dizziness, unsteadiness, nausea
Lamotrigine (Lamictal)	Dizziness, headaches, double vision, coordination problems

may be helpful. Capsaicin is the chemical that gives hot peppers, like jalapenos, their spicy kick. When applied to the skin, capsaicin depletes the nerve endings of the chemical they need to relay painful sensory information to the spinal cord. Another effective topical treatment may be to apply an ice pack for a few minutes to a painful area. Lidocaine patches are also often useful for relieving nerve pain. For painful dysesthesias that do not respond to any of the treatments discussed above, other interventions such as medications or a referral to a pain management specialist may be helpful.

Another type of dysesthesia brought on by demyelination in the cervical spinal cord (neck) is called L'hermitte's sign. Seen in about 25% to 40% of people with MS, it announces itself as a series of electric-buzzing-type sensations—ranging from odd to painful—that radiate down the spine and/or into the arms or legs when the neck is flexed forward. This symptom may be present for weeks to months and then disappear, only to spontaneously reappear sometime in the future. While this symptom can be alarming and uncomfortable, it's important to note that no new damage is caused by flexing the neck when this symptom is present.

Yet another dysesthesia is **trigeminal neuralgia**—facial pain, sometimes quite intense, that travels along one of the three branches of the trigeminal nerve, which supplies sensation to the face. The trigeminal nerve has three main branches (ophthalmic, maxillary, and mandibular) that provide sensation to the upper, middle, and lower portions of the face, respectively.

Trigeminal neuralgia is also known as tic douloureux and causes intense, electric shock–like pains that may last seconds or minutes. The pain most commonly involves the lower branch of the trigeminal nerve, resulting in pain in the lower face, and may be provoked by chewing or even a light touch to the face.

Nerve pain such as trigeminal neuralgia does not respond well to conventional pain medicines, such as those taken for a headache or for a broken bone. Rather, pain like trigeminal neuralgia must be treated with antiseizure medications that can settle down the increased nerve signaling in the CNS that is causing the pain.

Typically carbamazepine, oxcarbazepine, or gabapentin are used to treat this pain. Side effects may include dizziness, drowsiness, unsteadiness, and nausea. With carbamazepine and oxcarbazepine blood testing may be needed periodically to monitor for abnormalities of white blood cells and serum sodium.

While antiseizure medications are quite effective in treating trigeminal neuralgia, not everyone will respond, and the pain may persist. These cases of trigeminal neuralgia may need a surgical approach. Procedures to reduce the pain interrupt the signaling from the trigeminal nerve. A common procedure is to use radio frequency that will create a small lesion on the trigeminal nerve that interrupts the pain signal. Another procedure uses radiation with a specialized Gamma Knife to interrupt the pain signal. As with any surgical procedure, the risks and benefits should be discussed with the surgeon so that an informed decision can be made.

Occipital neuralgia causes pain in the distribution of the occipital nerve. The occipital nerve exits the base of the skull and supplies sensation to the scalp. Occipital neuralgia may result in pain ranging from dull to intense, sometimes with hypersensitivity to touch over the scalp. Occipital neuralgia is also treated with anticonvulsants like carbamazepine, oxcarbazepine, and gabapentin. Anti-inflammatory medications like indomethacin may also be helpful. Local injections at the base of the skull using steroids and anesthetic agents can be used to both treat and diagnose occipital neuralgia.

Summary

Sensory disturbances are common among people with MS. In some cases, they might not rise above the level of a nuisance. In other cases, however, they can cause real problems with tasks of daily life, including painful dysesthesia, trigeminal neuralgia, and occipital neuralgia. Treatment options exist for each of these symptoms, all of which require a neurologist's assessment before being explored.

Issues with Vision and Other Senses

Vision

Visual impairment is pretty common in MS. In about 15% of people with MS, the first symptom is an episode of optic neuritis (remember Susan in Chapter 1). Optic neuritis is a temporary loss of vision in one or both eyes that is often painful, and is caused by inflammation ("itis") of the optic nerve. Optic neuritis is commonly treated with a brief course of steroids and the person usually recovers full or at least functional vision in the affected eye. Other vision problems that may be caused by MS include blurry vision, double vision, or jumping vision (i.e., the world appears as though it is moving when it really is not). When vision problems are new or newly worsening and develop over several days, they may be considered an exacerbation or relapse of MS. In the absence of any infection, acute episodes of vision problems are generally treated with a short course of steroids (see Chapter 5).

Other Senses

While it is very uncommon for MS to cause problems with hearing, this occasionally happens. People may experience decreased hearing or ringing in the ears (i.e., tinnitus). Because hearing problems are so uncommon in MS, it is advisable to rule out other causes first before assuming the hearing problem is related to MS. It is even rarer for MS to cause difficulty with taste or smell, but once in a while people with MS will report unpleasant tastes or the inability to taste or smell. Again, it is a good idea to look for other causes of these symptoms because they are so unusual in MS. This and other symptoms should be discussed with your neurologist so that the appropriate investigations can be undertaken and the best treatment plan developed.

How Multiple Sclerosis Can Affect Memory and Other Cognitive Functions

All of us have moments of forgetfulness from time to time. It is normal, for example, to misplace your keys, to walk into a room and suddenly forget why you are there, or to have trouble finding certain commonplace words during a conversation. So what distinguishes such everyday lapses from the kinds of memory and other cognitive difficulties experienced by some people with MS?

Most people with MS never have severe intellectual difficulties. Mild problems, however, are relatively common. About 60% of people with MS experience a change in some area of cognitive function, with memory being the one most typically affected. Approximately 80% of those people will have mild deficits, and about 10% to 20% report moderate or severe ones. While MS can cause cognitive difficulties, other factors can also contribute to cognitive symptoms, including fatigue, poor sleep, pain, medication side effects, and depression. These factors must also be addressed when cognitive symptoms are identified.

Let's look at three patient stories illustrating a range of MS-related cognitive symptoms, from mild to moderate to severe.

> Donald was diagnosed with MS 17 years ago and is now 52 years old. He is a pharmacist at a busy teaching hospital and works with several research projects examining new cancer therapies.
>
> *(Continued)*

(Continued)

Generally, his MS has been well controlled with no relapses for years, but he has begun to notice some mild difficulty remembering the multiple steps involved in some research protocols, and sometimes he needs to refer back to the written instructions. His treating neurologist orders a full battery of cognitive tests that reveal a mild impairment in his ability to learn and remember new information, but not to the degree that would impact Donald's ability to work. Compensatory strategies that he is already using, such as referring to written protocols or instructions, help to keep him on track.

Rachel was diagnosed with MS 20 years ago and is now 46 years old. She works as a schoolteacher. Her school district has instituted a new curriculum and, because of budget cuts, has increased class sizes. Rachel finds it increasingly difficult to plan for her classroom activities. Her neurologist refers her to a **neuropsychologist** for a battery of cognitive tests. The tests reveal moderate problems with attention, speed of processing information, and the ability to learn new information. Based on these results and her neurologist's recommendations, the school district agrees to provide Rachel with a classroom assistant and to limit her class size.

Maurice is a 63-year-old man with MS since age 24. His course has been one of slowly progressive problems with walking for the past 18 years. He is unable to walk and has frequent bladder accidents. His family cannot leave him

(Continued)

(Continued)
alone for any period of time because he acts out impulsively. In the doctor's waiting room he makes inappropriate comments about other people, including the neurologist's nurse. A complete workup by his neurologist shows no explanation for this behavior other than his MS.

Cognitive function encompasses areas that, in addition to memory, include attention, concentration, speed of thought, information processing, problem solving, and judgment.

Attention and concentration are subtly different. Attention refers to the state of being aware and generally focused. Concentration refers to being focused on a specific task. Each of these is a key component of cognitive function, and they are interwoven and influenced by a number of factors. Memory is a highly complex multistep process that involves learning information, storing and organizing information, and retrieving information when it is needed. Multiple sclerosis principally affects short-term memory. That is, a person with MS might have trouble remembering a phone number learned in the past couple of months but will likely recall facts learned in the distant past—for instance, the multiplication tables. In order to perform well, memory needs nerve fiber pathways that function normally. Since those pathways are in varying degrees damaged and obstructed by MS, the storage, organization, and retrieval of information can be impaired.

Multiple sclerosis particularly affects the type of short-term memory known as working memory. Working memory helps the mind temporarily store and manage information needed for learning, reasoning, and comprehension. Many routine tasks, such as turning off the oven, knowing where the keys are, or recalling a phone number, involve working memory. Having mild working-memory problems can be frustrating, and more moderate problems will interfere with daily life, as seen in our earlier cases.

Multiple sclerosis can also have an impact on other cognitive areas, including thought-processing speed, attention, concentration, and **executive function** (see below). Impairments in these areas of cognitive functioning can also influence how well or poorly working memory performs. People experiencing slower thought-processing speed often describe feeling frustrated when they are unable to respond to a question as quickly as they once could. They may become anxious when a bit of information they need is not readily recalled. Others describe difficulty concentrating on a task, particularly when there are distractions—for instance, a conversation going on within earshot or the noise of a TV in the next room. Worse, job performance can be hampered by such changes in cognitive function. An individual may find that he or she can no longer keep up with the workload or the pace of the job.

John was diagnosed with MS 10 years ago and is now 37 years old. He has been working in sales for 15 years, and over the past year has found it difficult to keep up with all of his accounts. He used to be able to keep all account information in his head and had the ability to retrieve the information at will. Now he finds that if he does not write something down, he cannot remember it. Also, if he tries to retrieve account information from his head, he mixes up his different accounts. He must now refer to his computer to provide accurate information and is able to compensate for his difficulties with memory and mental organization, but it is a laborious process that takes a lot of time—so much so that he is losing sales and having difficulty keeping pace with the other sales associates. He is fearful that these difficulties will cost him his job.

Executive function is the cognitive area that includes reasoning, organizing, prioritizing, decision-making, and problem solving. It, too, can be affected in MS. Executive function is important for planning, particularly when a plan needs to be suddenly changed based on new information—for example, if your daily train has been cancelled, and you need to find new transportation home. It is also the function that enables people to shift or divide attention. Finally, executive function acts as a brake on impulsive behavior and is responsible for keeping us from acting socially inappropriate. When this "brake" is lost the person is said to be "disinhibited."

Cognitive dysfunction as a result of MS often disrupts fluency and produces the "tip-of-the-tongue" experience; some people with MS notice that when they want to say a familiar word, they can't find it.

We met Rachel and Maurice earlier. Rachel has moderate cognitive dysfunction, while Maurice's is more severe. Rachel's problems with executive functioning manifest as difficulty focusing on the task at hand without distractions, and she needs to develop strategies to enable her to focus. For instance, if she's grading papers at home, she needs to turn her cell phone off and make sure her husband is playing with the children in another room. Maurice, because of his more severe cognitive symptoms, shows executive dysfunction by exhibiting disinhibited behavior. Maurice makes inappropriate comments about people including nurses in the neurologist's office.

Evaluating and Treating Cognitive Function Difficulties

Neuropsychologists are the healthcare providers who evaluate cognitive function. They rely on special tests that have been developed to determine whether problems in different areas of thinking, or cognitive domains, exist. These tests help identify cognitive strengths as well as limitations. They consist of a variety of tasks designed to measure various cognitive abilities. A full neuropsychological battery can take 7 to 8 hours. It is typically divided into two or more shorter sessions because some people become fatigued. The neuropsychologist will initiate the neurocognitive assessment with a detailed interview to evaluate whether stress, depression, medications (notably, ones that produce sedation, such as some pain-killers), fatigue, or physical symptoms might be contributing to difficulties with concentration and memory.

Assessing cognitive function requires a battery of different tests. Although the specific tests may vary with different neuropsychologists, there will be some similarities. The neuropsychologist will use different tests to assess common cognitive domains, such as the ones discussed above, namely, working and short-term memory, attention, judgment, recall, and executive function.

Currently, there are no medications that treat cognitive problems caused by MS. Clinical trials in MS of the drugs used to treat the memory problems associated with Alzheimer's disease were not definitively found to be helpful, although sometimes they are still tried with varying degrees of success. The use of these medications does not suggest any similarity between the pathology of Alzheimer's and MS. The medications are intended to help with the symptom of impaired memory, not to treat the underlying disease process.

Once specific areas of cognitive difficulty have been identified through neuropsychological testing, however, a number of cognitive retraining strategies can be introduced. For example, someone with executive function difficulties could work with a neuropsychologist to develop a more structured daily routine that includes techniques to help the person focus on one task at a time and to filter out distractions when attention and concentration are the problem. Several research studies have recently been conducted to evaluate the benefits of different cognitive retraining strategies in people with MS. These have yielded some promising results showing improved recall in some cases. However, more research in this area is needed.

People with MS who experience cognitive difficulties can find the experience upsetting and at times even frightening. As with any physical symptoms, it is important to discuss cognitive symptoms with your doctors so that the symptoms can be thoroughly investigated and management strategies, which in the case of cognitive difficulties may include self-directed strategies, can be developed and implemented.

Genitourinary Problems

Genitourinary (GU) problems refer to dysfunction of the bladder, bowel, and sexual function. While GU symptoms are common in MS, most problems can be effectively managed with lifestyle modifications and/or medications.

Bladder Symptoms

Bladder symptoms are common in MS, affecting about three out of four of people with MS. The usual symptoms of bladder dysfunction are urgency frequency, hesitancy, and incontinence (leakage or loss of bladder control).

The bladder is like a big bag with a muscular wall. Its job is to stretch and fill with urine that comes from both kidneys. Normally, the receptors in the bladder are able to detect when about a cup of urine is present and then send a "full" signal to the spinal cord. That signal travels up to the brain, where it is interpreted and if the timing is appropriate, an outgoing message is sent back to the bladder telling it to contract. At the same time, a message is given to the sphincter muscle (which controls the opening out of the bladder), allowing it to relax and permit urine to flow. Both involuntary activity and voluntary activity are involved with bladder function. For instance, even though the signal that the bladder is full may be sent, the moment may not be optimal for urination. If you're in a meeting and can't get to the bathroom, your brain sends signals to "hold" the urine until there is a better opportunity for urination.

In MS, several problems may arise that interfere with bladder function. These problems can be categorized into three areas: difficulty with urine storage in the bladder, difficulty with emptying the bladder, and a disconnect between the bladder contractions and the sphincter activity.

Difficulty with Urine Storage

Difficulty with urine storage is the most common elimination problem in MS. Sometimes the signal that the bladder should be emptied occurs long before the bladder is full, leading to the need to urinate frequently. These abnormal bladder contractions produce a number of symptoms including urgency, frequency, and sometimes urgency incontinence (loss of bladder control due to urgency).

Management includes monitoring the intake of known bladder irritants such as caffeine, artificial sweeteners, and alcoholic beverages, and frequent timed voiding. In addition, a number of medications can be used to reduce bladder overactivity, and these are often very effective treatments.

Difficulty with Bladder Emptying

Sometimes the bladder fills and the signal to empty is disrupted somewhere along the spinal cord or brain pathways. This disruption may produce a bladder that holds too much urine and does not empty adequately. Symptoms may also include urgency and frequency. In addition, the person may experience a loss of bladder control, and bladder infections may occur as urine stays in the bladder too long. Emptying problems can sometimes be treated with medication and sometimes with a procedure called intermittent self-catheterization. While very few individuals will be excited to self-catheterize and the procedure sounds very complicated, it is actually a relatively simple procedure that requires the introduction of a small tube (catheter) through the urethra and into the bladder to mechanically empty the bladder. In someone with bladder-emptying difficulties, this procedure can often take care of the problem and alleviate the symptoms of urgency, frequency, or loss of control. Self-catheterizing may be done from one to several times/day based on individual need.

Difficulty with Detrusor/Sphincter Dyssynergia

Multiple sclerosis can cause difficulty with functions involving the detrusor, a bladder muscle, and the sphincter. These functions become discoordinated (i.e., dyssynergic), which results in an overactive bladder muscle that cannot empty itself against a nonrelaxed sphincter. Difficulty with detrusor/sphincter dyssynergia (DSD) produces symptoms of urgency, frequency, and incontinence and may also result in frequent bladder infections. Because DSD is a problem of both storage and emptying, treatment usually involves strategies to help calm down the overactive detrusor and simultaneously empty the bladder, for example, medication plus self-catheterization.

When symptoms of bladder dysfunction are present, your neurologist may recommend an evaluation with a urologist (a specialist in urinary function) to determine the specific problem, which will also help to determine the correct treatment. Testing with a urologist is called urodynamic testing. In this type of testing a catheter (thin tube) is inserted into the bladder. Fluid is introduced into the bladder through the catheter, and measurements of the pressures in the bladder and when the need to empty the bladder occurs are made. The amount of urine eliminated is also measured, as well as any urine that may remain in the bladder, which is called residual. This testing identifies the bladder function problem, and the correct treatment can then be prescribed.

Bowel symptoms

Bowel problems are very common among people with MS. Constipation is the usual bowel problem. Constipation may result from the nerve damage caused by MS as well as many other factors. These other factors may include decreased mobility, poor diet and fluid intake, and side effects from medications. Useful strategies to help improve bowel function include drinking plenty of noncaffeinated fluids; eating foods rich in fiber, such as fruits, vegetables, whole grains, and nuts; and increasing physical activity. Sometimes additional help with a stool softener, or suppository, is needed to facilitate a bowel movement at least three to four times a week. Laxatives may be used occasionally but should be avoided as a routine remedy. Their use should be discussed with a doctor, as many types of laxatives are available and some that are harsh bowel irritants should be avoided. Bowel symptoms should be discussed with the neurologist before any laxatives or enemas are used. In cases of bowel dysfunction that do not respond to the above measures, a consult with a gastroenterologist may be needed.

Sexual Dysfunction

Sexual dysfunction is also common among both men and women with MS. Possible symptoms can include erectile dysfunction, impaired ejaculation, reduced vaginal lubrication, difficulty experiencing orgasm, painful intercourse, and decreased libido. Side effects of certain medications commonly used in MS, including antidepressants, can contribute to sexual dysfunction. Unfortunately, too often a "don't ask, don't tell" stigma prevents these issues from being discussed openly. Some symptoms of sexual dysfunction respond well to treatments such as medication, lubricants, hormone replacement, devices, and specific intervention by a sex therapist. Your doctor may refer you to a urologist, gynecologist, or psychologist to assist in managing these symptoms.

Erectile dysfunction (ED), or the failure to achieve and maintain an erection, is common in the general population and can have several different causes. In men with MS it is caused by interference with the nerve signals necessary for arousal and erection. Evaluation of erectile dysfunction is best undertaken by a urologist who is familiar with MS. The evaluation of ED should include investigation for other conditions such as diabetes and medications that are known to affect sexual function such as certain antidepressants. Often ED in MS is successfully treated with medication such as sildenafil (Viagra) or tadalafil (Cialis). Other methods include drugs that are delivered directly into the penis, either by injection or suppository, or mechanical devices such as plastic implants or pumps. Both women and men can have difficulty reaching orgasm, a condition called anorgasmia. In women with MS this can occur from a variety of causes including nerve signal disruption in the brainstem or spinal cord, psychological issues, and emotional issues. In addition, certain medications can contribute to the problem including certain antidepressants and anticonvulsant medications. Treatments such as methods to enhance sensory stimulation to the genitals may be used.

Decreased libido in both men and women with MS may have many causes. It certainly can be a symptom of the MS itself, but may also be a result of depression, fatigue, pain, or other MS symptoms, and can also be caused by some medications. Most men and women with MS have normal hormone levels, but low levels of these can also cause decreased libido. A gynecologist or urologist consult is helpful in diagnosing and treating this problem.

While MS can cause primary sexual dysfunction as described above, other MS symptoms may contribute to difficulty in having satisfying sexual relations. These secondary causes might include fatigue, spasticity, bladder problems, or impaired or painful sensation to the genital area to name a few. These can all be successfully treated, so it is important to discuss this with your neurologist.

Summary

This chapter illustrates how the complexities of MS can produce many symptoms that can impact daily life, although it is unlikely that all of the symptoms discussed here will affect any one individual. While it is easy to attribute any symptom to MS, other causes are possible. Therefore, it is important to discuss all symptoms with the doctor so that the cause can be correctly identified and the appropriate treatment initiated. Treatment of symptoms in MS usually involves medications, rehabilitation, and lifestyle modification for optimal management. Persistence with a treatment plan—and modification of the treatment plan if needed—can greatly improve or ameliorate almost all of these problems and facilitate normal functioning and improved quality of life.

Chapter 5 discusses therapies that may alter the course of MS as well as recent research that is focused on this goal. Nevertheless, the importance of symptom management in MS cannot be overlooked. Managing the daily symptoms of MS can result in an immediate improvement in quality of life. Because of the wide range of symptoms, their fluctuating nature, and the multitude of treatment options, a partnership between the person with MS and their healthcare team needs to be in place.

Chapter 5

Treating and Managing Multiple Sclerosis

Relapses and Disease-Modifying Therapies

In this chapter, you'll learn:

- **What a relapse is**
- **How relapses are treated**
- **What disease-modifying therapies are and what do they do**

Relapses

As we learned in Chapter 1, most people with MS are initially diagnosed with the relapsing-remitting form of the disease. Admittedly, the term "relapsing-remitting" can be a little misleading. Normally, the word "remission" means a period of being symptom-free. While recovery from a relapse occurs, it can be incomplete, with some persistence of residual symptoms. Thus many people with MS are never entirely without symptoms. Usually, *something* is going on, be it fatigue, bladder problems, spasticity, or some other continuing symptom of the condition. And just to make things a bit more confusing, the ongoing, everyday symptoms, such as fatigue, may be worse on some days than on others. Factors such as sleep difficulties, stress, other illnesses, and heat exposure may determine whether one is having a good day or not. In MS terms, remission means a period of stability, with no intensifying symptoms or acute attacks.

True Relapses

"Attack." "Exacerbation." "Flare-up." These are all terms used to describe the "relapsing" part of relapsing-remitting MS. How does someone know if a relapse is occurring? A relapse is defined as new or newly worsening neurological symptoms that last greater than 24 hours and not being provoked by a metabolic issue such as a fever or infection. An example of a relapse could be the new onset of visual blurring that develops over several days.

Rachel is a 41-year-old woman who has had relapsing-remitting MS for the past 8 years. She is the leader of a support group for people with MS. At their last support group meeting, two newly diagnosed individuals were in attendance. Both asked the question, "How will we know if we are having a relapse?" Rachel used examples from her own medical history to help explain.

"One of my earliest MS symptoms was numbness in both legs," Rachel began. "It improved after a few weeks but never went away completely. About 2 years ago, the numbness suddenly began to get worse and now went up a little higher on my legs. After 2 days of this, I called my neurologist. He took my history, did an exam, and made sure that I did not have an infection, such as a bladder infection. My neurologist then told me that this counted as an exacerbation. I was treated with 3 days of intravenous steroids, and after the second dose, my symptoms improved to their prior baseline."

Rachel went on to describe another episode from about 9 years ago. "We were at the beach for a summer trip. I woke up with pain around my left eye and noticed that things

(Continued)

(Continued)

seemed blurry in that eye. I called my neurologist and saw her as soon as we got home. She told me I had optic neuritis. I got a course of steroids, and after about 3 weeks the vision was back to normal."

When Is a Relapse Not a Relapse?

You might think that the occurrence of a relapse should be obvious. Sometimes it is, and sometimes it isn't. A person can experience a new or worsened neurologic symptom due to overexertion or becoming overheated or due to an infection (such as a cold or a bladder infection). This is called a **pseudo-exacerbation**. With pseudo-exacerbations, the symptoms are real, but the underlying cause is something besides MS. Symptoms that worsen due to heat or exercise usually diminishes within hours. It is important to understand that heat and overexertion do not cause new MS lesions to form, nor do they create permanent nerve fiber damage. Symptoms that worsen during an infection will typically improve when the infection subsides or is treated. In other words, a pseudo-exacerbation is a relapse that can be attributed to a known cause such as an infection or rise in body temperature.

John is a 53-year-old man who has had relapsing-remitting MS for 20 years. For the past 5 years, he has done very well, with no relapses. Over the course of a few days, he notices that he needs to urinate much more frequently and that his urine appears cloudy. John also has some mild burning

(Continued)

(Continued)

with urination. At the same time, he also notices weakness in both legs and an increase in painful muscle spasms. John usually gets around with the help of a cane, but now he needs to use a rolling walker. He sees his neurologist, and a urinalysis confirms a bladder infection. John's doctor explains that this infection is likely causing the worsened neurologic symptoms, and that this is called a pseudo-exacerbation. After a course of oral antibiotics, John's symptoms resolve.

Dealing with the Impact of Relapses

Clearly, relapses are key events in MS. With each one, there is a chance that some of the new or worsened symptoms can become permanent. Unfortunately, currently no reliable methods exist to predict when the symptoms of a relapse will recede with time and when they are here to stay.

The goal of long-term disease-modifying therapy in MS is to reduce the frequency of relapses or prevent them altogether. **Disease-modifying therapies**, for MS or any other disease, are those that actually modify the underlying mechanism of the disease itself, rather than just temporarily alleviating symptoms. It is important that people who have MS tell their physicians when relapses happen. The frequency and severity of relapses, as well as recovery from them, all play a role in deciding whether to continue with a particular disease-modifying therapy or to try another one. The physician may also help to determine whether the event is a relapse due to MS or a pseudo-relapse.

Relapses in MS do matter. Research by Dr. Fred Lublin, director of the Corinne Goldsmith Dickinson Center for Multiple Sclerosis at Mt. Sinai Hospital in New York, showed that with each MS relapse, there is about a 28% chance of significant persistent worsening of neurologic functioning 2 months after the relapse. Another study showed that people who experienced more relapses in the first 2 years after an MS diagnosis needed to use a cane earlier than those with fewer relapses that occurred during this time.

While it is important to keep physicians notified about relapses, it may not be necessary for physicians to treat all of them. Research has shown that treatment may speed recovery from a relapse. However, the degree of recovery, with or without treatment, appears to be the same. In other words, treatment enables patients to reach the same point of recovery as they would without treatment, but more quickly. Ultimately, the decision about whether to seek relapse-management treatment depends on how troublesome the relapse symptoms are, that is, how much they interfere with your ability to carry out your usual activities. Other factors that must be considered are the side effects and risks of relapse treatment, other health problems that could cause problems with a particular treatment, and the history of the individual patient's response to previous relapse treatments.

Treatments to Manage Relapses

Most commonly, relapses are treated with high doses of glucocorticoids, which are types of steroids that are anti-inflammatory drugs, not the kinds of steroids used by body builders. Since MS is an inflammatory process, as we've discussed in previous chapters, reducing inflammation can help alleviate MS symptoms. Steroids are very good at treating the symptoms of a relapse and helping them to resolve more quickly, but they have not been shown to alter the long-term course of MS.

Steroids are usually given intravenously (into a vein, or IV) or by mouth. Methylprednisolone (Solu-Medrol) is the IV steroid used most often, although dexamethasone (Decadron) is also employed.

Methylprednisolone is generally given intravenously in doses of 500 to 1,000 milligrams per day for 3 to 5 days. Prednisone is an oral steroid that may be taken after IV steroids are administered, with the dosage gradually reduced over time. This period of gradual reduction in the prednisone dose typically lasts 1 to 2 weeks, and then the prednisone is stopped all together. Many people with MS do well using IV steroids alone with no prednisone given. Another steroid option for relapse management is high-dose prednisone (600 mg to 1,250 mg) taken by mouth for 3 to 5 days. As with intravenous steroids, the dosage may or may not be reduced gradually. This regimen is used more frequently in Canada than in the United States. Studies suggest that the benefits and side effects of IV and oral steroids are similar. You may ask your doctor to give you oral steroids because you do not like receiving regular injections, or you may find that you experience more side effects with an oral drug and prefer to be given steroids by IV. Your doctor may also have specific recommendations about which method to use, depending on your individual circumstances.

Here are some ways of thinking through a possible relapse and its management:

1. If you have new or worsened neurologic symptoms lasting more than 24 hours,* is there an explanation other than MS? (*Please note that it's okay to contact your doctor for new or worsened symptoms prior to 24 hours for advice.)
2. If the symptoms are considered to be attributable to an underlying infection, treat that infection appropriately.
3. If the symptoms are thought to be the result of a relapse, discuss whether to treat with steroids. This will depend on how bothersome the symptoms are. Are there reasons you should not be treated with steroids? These might include a history of steroid side effects or health problems that may make steroid treatment less safe, such as uncontrolled hypertension or diabetes mellitus. Remember, treatment with steroids

may speed up recovery but does not change the degree of recovery. It may be okay to just watch and let the symptoms improve.

4. If the symptoms are bothersome enough to treat with steroids (i.e., severe enough to interfere with your usual functions), the doctor will discuss with you what type of steroids to consider and how long you might need to take them. No strict guidelines exist, and some of this will depend on your individual history and the doctor's preference. Options include:

   a. Three to 5 days of intravenous methylprednisolone with or without an oral steroid taper afterward.

   b. Short regimens of various oral steroids, for example, dexamethasone or prednisone

   c. Alternatives to intravenous or oral steroids, to be discussed below.

Nonsteroid treatments employed to help manage exacerbations include intravenous immunoglobulin (IVIg), adrenocorticotropic hormone (ACTH), and plasma exchange.

Intravenous immunoglobulin is a solution of human antibodies that, typically, is given intravenously over the course of 5 days. Potential side effects of IVIg include headaches, fever, muscle aches, and the possibility of contracting blood-borne infections, such as hepatitis. More serious, but less common side effects include aseptic meningitis (inflammation around the lining of the brain with no actual infection), blood clots in the legs or lungs, and kidney dysfunction.

Adrenocorticotropic hormone is a human hormone that stimulates the body to produce natural steroids, which, like the artificial steroids described above, can minimize the inflammatory process associated with MS relapses. Traditionally, ACTH is given by daily injection directly into the muscle over a 2-week period. More recent research has suggested that ACTH can be given daily for 5 days by a shallower subcutaneous injection, to treat relapses. Even though

ACTH is not itself a steroid, it does lead to the increased production of natural steroids. Therefore, the side effects of ACTH are similar to those of steroids.

Plasma exchange (or plasmapheresis) is a procedure used to filter out antibodies in the blood stream that are causing inflammation. Side effects from plasma exchange include infections, electrolyte (blood chemical) imbalances, and blood-clotting problems.

Generally, IVIg, ACTH, and plasma exchange are employed in situations in which the patient cannot tolerate or has not responded to steroid therapy.

As suggested, the potential benefits of steroid therapy must be weighed against the risk of side effects. For example, steroids may bring about mood changes; a person can veer from feeling energized and euphoric to feeling agitated and anxious. Sometimes that anxiety can lead to trouble getting to sleep while on the steroids. In some people, steroids spur an increase in stomach acid production (resulting in heartburn or indigestion). Steroids may stimulate the appetite and produce weight gain. They often cause fluid retention. The steroids also carry a risk of temporarily increased blood pressure or blood sugar production, meaning that people with hypertension or diabetes need to be monitored when steroids are given. If necessary, doses of insulin can be given to correct elevations of blood sugar caused by steroids in people with diabetes. Long-term use of steroids can increase the risk of osteoporosis and cataracts.

Summary

Relapses are a basic feature of relapsing-remitting MS, the most common form of the disease. Relapses are usually treated when they interfere with a person's ability to carry out normal activities. The decision about whether to embark on relapse-management treatment hinges on the question of how much or how little trouble the relapse symptoms are causing. Relapses are most commonly treated with a brief course of oral or intravenous steroids; sometimes other treatments may also be used. Ongoing relapses may be an indication that a patient's disease-modifying therapy isn't working adequately. Recurrent relapses need to be addressed because they have the potential to cause increased long-term disability.

Disease-Modifying Therapies

At present there is no known cure for MS, but a number of approved medications can be used to manage its effects. They fall into three categories: (1) medications used to treat an acute relapse (described above); (2) medications used help manage MS symptoms (Chapter 4); and (3) medications used to interfere with the immune system's attack on the nervous system. The medications that make up the third category, known as disease-modifying therapies (DMTs), are the focus of the rest of this chapter.

As discussed in Chapter 1, MS is an autoimmune disorder, a condition in which the immune system misguidedly attacks myelin—the fatty material that insulates nerve fibers (axons) in the brain and spinal cord and facilitates the transmission of nerve impulses—as if it were a foreign invader rather than a normal part of the body. As a result, the myelin becomes inflamed, damaged, and in many cases destroyed. Scars (scleroses) form, and the axons themselves are damaged. This process slows and blocks the transmission of nerve impulses that are involved in muscle coordination, physical strength, sensation, vision, and cognition.

In MS, disease modification involves employing certain medications to slow or stop the destruction of myelin (demyelination) and resultant formation of scars (scleroses) on the nerves of the brain and spinal cord. Since antimyelin attacks are driven by the immune system, treatments that "modify" or change the course of MS are called immune modifiers or DMTs. Currently, no DMT has been shown to completely halt the progression of MS or completely stop all relapses for all—people with relapsing forms of MS. Various research studies that have looked at the natural history of MS, and those who have investigated the effects of the DMTs indicate that early intervention with a DMT is the best treatment strategy. For many people, this approach will reduce the number and severity of relapses and limit the damage that produces some of the progressive disability associated with MS.

How early should DMTs be considered in MS? The earliest sign of relapsing-remitting MS is the first attack. Someone with a first onset of neurologic symptoms that are consistent with MS is often diagnosed with a clinically isolated syndrome (CIS). If a person presents with a CIS and has brain MRI changes consistent with MS and/or abnormalities on their spinal fluid examination, they may have up to a 90% chance of going on to have another episode or new area of nerve damage appear on their MRI, and thus having MS diagnosed. Some of the DMTs administered following a CIS have been shown to delay the occurrence of the next neurological event by up to 2 years.

Infrequently some people with MS may follow a mild—or so-called benign—course without incurring many relapses or significant disability, even if they do not have treatment with DMTs. Unfortunately, there is no way to predict which people with MS will follow a benign course. Some doctors advocate a period of observation for the person with newly diagnosed MS to see whether he or she might do well without treatment. However, most doctors and researchers would argue that this is a risky approach and believe that it is safer to initiate a DMT in all newly diagnosed with MS, and those with CIS who are considered at high risk for conversion to MS.

The goals of therapy with DMTs are to reduce the number or severity of relapses, slow the progression of disability, and lessen the emergence of new areas of MS inflammatory activity that can be seen on MRI. They should be thought of as a future-oriented insurance policy, while symptom-managing medications (Chapter 4) are aimed at helping the person feel better in the present. It is vital to have realistic expectations for DMTs, that is, to understand that they can help lessen the number of MS flare-ups but cannot prevent them entirely.

Although effective drug therapies approved by the US Food and Drug Administration (FDA) are available to help modify the relapsing-remitting and progressive-relapsing forms of MS, treatment options for the secondary-progressive or primary-progressive courses of the disease are less well defined. Remember also that the transition from relapsing-remitting MS to secondary-progressive MS is not a sudden leap. People with secondary-progressive MS can still have relapses and may benefit from the use of a DMT.

David visits his neurologist for his regularly scheduled follow-up MS evaluation.

"That new drug, Copaxone, isn't working," he tells his doctor, "I don't feel any better and I'm still having the same symptoms!"

The doctor says, "Let's back up a bit. Are you having any relapses?" David indicates he has not. "Are there any new or worsened symptoms?" Again, David says there are not. "Well, that's great!" his neurologist tells him. "And remember those recent MRIs we did? They showed you don't have any new MS lesions or inflammation. And the results of your neurologic examination today are the same as they were a year ago. So the DMT we're using is doing everything we had hoped. Now, let's talk about those symptoms you're still experiencing and how we might manage them."

By the mid-2010s, 12 DMTs had been approved by the FDA for the treatment of MS. Table 5–1 lists of all the FDA-approved DMTs.

TABLE 5-1 US Food and Drug Administration–Approved Disease-Modifying Therapies for Multiple Sclerosis

Medication	Route of Administration	Frequency	Common Side Effects
Betaseron/ Extavia	Subcutaneous injection	Every other day	Flulike symptoms, depression, headache, blood count and liver abnormalities, injection site reactions
Avonex	Intramuscular injection	Weekly	Flulike symptoms, depression, headache, blood count and liver abnormalities, injection site reactions
Rebif	Subcutaneous injection	3 times a week	Flulike symptoms, depression, headache, blood count and liver abnormalities, injection site reactions
Plegridy	Subcutaneous injection	Every 2 weeks	Same side effects as the other beta interferons
Copaxone	Subcutaneous injection	Daily or 3 times a week	Injection site reactions
Novantrone	Intravenous	Up to once a month	Blood count and liver abnormalities, cardiac damage, leukemia, infertility, infection
Tysabri	Intravenous	Once a month	Blood count and liver abnormalities, progressive multifocal leukoencephalopathy

TABLE 5-1 Continued

Medication	Route of Administration	Frequency	Common Side Effects
Gilenya	Oral	Daily	Cardiac problems, infection, blood count and liver abnormalities, infection
Aubagio	Oral	Daily	blood count and liver abnormalities, infection, hair loss (usually temporary)
Tecfidera	Oral	Twice a day	Nausea, abdominal pain, diarrhea, blood count and liver abnormalities, infection (one case of progressive multifocal leukeoencephalopathy)
Lemtrada	Intravenous	Once yearly	Blood count abnormalities, risk of other autoimmune diseases, infections, infusion reactions

The first DMT to be approved by the FDA was a brand of beta interferon called Betaseron. There are three major types of human interferons. The ones that MS DMTs replicate are called beta interferons. The others are alpha interferons, which can be synthesized for use in cancer and hepatitis treatment, and gamma interferons, which the immune system employs to increase inflammation.

Beta Interferons

Interferons were first identified in 1957, and investigations of beta interferon, a naturally occurring protein that helps the body fight infection and control the immune system, for use in MS therapy began not long afterward. Testing indicated that it showed some promise in slowing the progression of MS. However, it was difficult to obtain sufficient amounts of this protein to treat large numbers of patients. The introduction of recombinant DNA technology allowed scientists to clone, modify, and stabilize the beta interferon gene. This breakthrough, which took place in 1980, made it possible to manufacture beta interferon in sizable quantities. Beta interferon works in MS in part by diminishing the production of inflammatory chemicals (cytokines) and the number of inflammatory immune cells, as well as altering the ability of these immune cells to enter the brain.

Avonex, Betaseron, Extavia, Rebif, and Plegridy are all genetically engineered copies of interferon-beta. Plegridy also has the addition of another molecule that makes it longer acting. Although these therapies are administered with different frequency and by different types of injections, all work similarly in the body. Avonex is injected into the muscle (intramuscularly), by the patient, once a week. Those who use Betaseron or Extavia self-inject under the skin (subcutaneously) every other day. Rebif is subcutaneously self-injected 3 times a week. Plegridy is administered by subcutaneous injection once every 2 weeks. All of the interferons have an available auto-injector, a spring-loaded device into which the syringe of medication can be loaded. The injection is then given with the simple push of a button.

Beta interferon has several potential side effects. Among these are flulike symptoms that arise after self-injection; these symptoms usually lessen over the first few weeks of starting the drug. Starting with a partial dose and titrating to the full dose over several weeks may help keep these side effects to a minimum. Taking acetaminophen (Tylenol), ibuprofen (Motrin, Advil), or naproxen (Aleve) before injection is also helpful. Injection site reactions, including redness, mild swelling, and discomfort, may occur, particularly with the subcutaneously administered interferons. In addition, changes in the results of blood count (lowered white blood cell counts most commonly) or elevations of liver function tests may occur while beta interferon is being used, so blood levels should be monitored periodically during the course of therapy. Other possible side effects of beta interferon include headaches and depression. Sometimes women may experience irregular menstrual cycles.

Beta interferon has been approved by the FDA for the treatment of MS patients with relapsing forms of the disease or for people presenting with a CIS and high risk for future attacks. It is important to realize that beta interferons do not reverse the damage that has already occurred and will not relieve current symptoms. Some people can develop antibodies to beta interferon, which may reduce its effectiveness.

Glatiramer Acetate

Another early DMT, glatiramer acetate (Copaxone), is an injectable DMT used for those with relapsing-remitting MS and people with a CIS and a high risk for future attacks. Copaxone consists of four amino acids (glutamic acid, lysine, alanine, and tyrosine) combined to create a molecule that resembles a component of myelin called myelin basic protein. In early experiments with this compound, scientists sought to produce an MS-like illness called experimental allergic encephalomyelitis (EAE) in laboratory animals. Surprisingly, Copaxone blocked, rather than caused, the development of EAE. That serendipitous discovery led to clinical trials of this drug with patients with MS that proved to be effective. Since the compound looks similar to myelin basic protein, it was initially thought to act as a decoy, drawing the immune attack toward itself rather than toward the brain and spinal cord. While that indeed may be part of how Copaxone works, it also seems that the medication shifts the immune system away from the inflammatory state and toward a more anti-inflammatory state.

Copaxone is subcutaneously self-injected once a day (as a 20-mg dose) or 3 times per week (as a 40-mg dose), Its most common side effects are redness, itching, pain, or lumps that form at the sites of injections; generally, these reactions subside over weeks of usage. Less commonly, a post-injection reaction may occur, characterized by brief feelings of tightness of the chest, shortness of breath, sweating, and, sometimes, nausea that occurs during or right after an injection. Although alarming, these reactions do not represent a serious health risk. Additionally, some people experience atrophy of the subcutaneous tissue in areas where Copaxone is repeatedly injected. Copaxone requires no laboratory monitoring.

Trials comparing the effectiveness of Copaxone to Rebif and Betaseron have shown similar effectiveness in reducing relapses between those brands of beta interferon, and glatiramer acetate. The decision to use a beta interferon versus Copaxone will depend on individual factors such as the presence of other health issues like liver problems, depression, or migraine headaches (which may be aggravated by beta interferon); prior treatment with DMTs; injection frequency; and other lifestyle issues, such as the ability to comply with the blood tests needed to monitor people taking beta interferon.

Together, the beta interferons and glatiramer acetate are referred to as the ABCREP drugs (Avonex, Betaseron, Copaxone, Rebif, Extavia, and Plegridy). Research has shown that they are more effective when started early in the course of the disease. Nonetheless, many people with relapsing forms of MS do not take any of them. Why not? Some of the reasons cited by people refusing these drugs include fear of injections and needles, fear of side effects, and concerns about cost of the medications. These can generally be addressed and overcome with support from peers, nurse trainers, and financial-assistance counselors. Financial assistance is widely available through the manufacturers of each medication.

Intravenous Medications

The FDA has approved three intravenous medications for use in MS disease modification. These are natalizumab (Tysabri), mitoxantrone (Novantrone), and alembuzumab (Lemtrada). Typically, the people who use them have not responded adequately or have had intolerable side effects to the ABCREP drugs.

Natalizumab (Tysabri), which is administered intravenously once a month, belongs to a class of drugs called monoclonal antibodies, which are immune proteins that are designed to influence certain steps in the immune process. Tysabri is indicated as monotherapy (not to be used with any other DMT) for relapsing forms of multiple sclerosis. Tysabri prevents immune system white blood cells from entering the brain by blocking their ability to attach to blood vessels there. This reduces the immune cells' ability to attack and damage myelin and axons in the CNS. Tysabri is administered in a medical clinic by personnel who have received training and approval to administer the mediation. An IV is placed with each visit, and the infusion itself takes about an hour. Another hour of observation is performed after the infusion. The drug was originally approved for first-line use in treating relapsing-remitting MS in 2004; however, it was withdrawn from the market early the following year after two people developed a potentially fatal viral brain infection called progressive multifocal leukoencephalopathy (PML). In both cases, PML occurred when Tysabri was combined with Avonex in clinical trials. After extensive investigation by regulatory authorities and the drug manufacturer, Tysabri was reintroduced in 2006. A safety-monitoring program was instituted at that time called Tysabri Outreach: Unified Commitment to Health (TOUCH) Prescribing Program. Progressive multifocal leukoencephalopathy has continued to occur since the relaunch of the drug, even when Tysabri is used by itself. Under the TOUCH Prescribing Program, every patient who receives Tysabri is closely monitored for the occurrence of PML and other serious infections, and the drug is immediately stopped if any such symptoms appear. Monitoring shows that PML is more likely to occur in people receiving Tysabri if certain conditions exist. For example, PML is caused by a virus known as the JC virus. Most people have been exposed to this virus at some time in their lives, and evidence of this exposure can be identified through a JC virus antibody test. Those who are JC virus antibody positive are at greater risk of developing PML. Also people who have been receiving Tysabri for more than 2 years are at greater risk of developing PML. Finally, individuals who have previously been treated with immune suppressants (such as cancer fighting drugs) are at greater risk of developing PML. Having more than one of these risk factors increases the risk even more. Thus, as with any drug, while effective, the risks of treatment need to be weighed against the expected benefits for each individual.

Tysabri is generally considered for use in cases of ongoing relapses or in those where, despite the use of ABCREP drugs, evidence of new MS activity has appeared on MRIs.

Mitoxantrone (Novantrone) is an immune suppressant that was first developed as a chemotherapy drug for certain cancers, including prostate cancer. It is employed for treatment in cases where aggressive types of relapsing-remitting or progressive MS persist despite ABCREP therapy. Typically, it is administered intravenously once every 3 months for up to 2 years. A serious side effect of Novanrone is that its use can produce heart damage. This risk increases when a certain total lifetime dose of the drug has been exceeded. Because of this concern, an echocardiogram or multigated acquisition (MUGA) scan is administered in order to monitor cardiac function before each dose is given, and even after the person is no longer taking Novantrone. These tests can measure the volume of blood being pumped by the heart with each beat. In addition, blood is tested after each Novantrone dose to gauge the transient and expected reduction in the white blood cell count. Monitoring is important because an increased risk of infection exists if the number of white blood cells drops too low. Leukemia has been reported as a result of Novantrone use and appears to be more common than was suspected in early trials. Novantrone can also cause permanent infertility. Given the availability of other options and the risks of cardiac damage and leukemia, Novantrone is being used far less frequently than in the past for MS.

Aletuzumab (Lemtrada) is a monoclonal antibody designed to deplete the numbers of certain types of white blood cells known as lymphocytes, including those lymphocytes believed to be important in MS inflammation and damage. Lemtrada is given by intravenous infusion once daily for 5 consecutive days and one year later for 3 consecutive days. Lemtrada has a number of serious and potentially fatal side effects and risks associated with its use. Infusion reactions (symptoms occurring during and even 24 hours or more after the infusion) are common. Treatment with IV steroids on the first 3 days of Lemtrada treatments is used to limit these reactions. Other longer term side effects include a greater risk of infections, other serious autoimmune diseases that can affect the thyroid or the kidney. Lemtrada has been known to provoke a serious bleeding disorder. There is also an increased risk for the development of certain cancers.

Due to theses serious side effects and risks, Lemtrada is recommended for use if someone has had an inadequate response to 2 other disease modifying treatments. It can only be administered in an approved infusion center. Monthly blood tests are required following the infusion of Lemtrada for at least 48 months.

When first-line agents (the ABCREP drugs) do not appear to be effective, several other drugs may be tried, one at a time. These drugs include steroids, immunoglobulin (IVIg), cyclophosphamide, methotrexate, azathioprine, and mycophenolate. The use of these drugs for disease modification is called "off label," meaning that they have not been approved by the FDA to treat MS, although they are approved to treat other diseases. In addition, the use of these drugs in various combinations is currently being researched with the goal of developing a greater number of DMT options for MS.

The question of how one defines an inadequate response can be challenging. An ideal response to any MS drug is when a person with MS experiences no relapses or progression of disability and when MRIs show that no new lesions or inflammation have occurred in the brain and/or spinal cord. However, the current therapies are not perfect. While many people with MS respond well to treatment, other people will continue to have relapses or progressive deficit no matter which drug is used. The decision to switch medications or stop them altogether depends on a number of factors, including the history of the person's compliance with the given drug, the risks and benefits of other treatment options, and the individual's personal preferences. In general, second-line options like natalizumab and mitoxantrone pose a greater risk of side effects than ABCREP therapies. People with MS will need to review these safety issues with their neurologist to determine which treatment course they are most comfortable with.

Oral Disease-Modifying Therapies

In September 2010, the FDA approved fingolimod (Gilenya) as the first oral DMT for relapsing forms of MS. As new treatment options become available, people with MS and healthcare providers will need to consider where these drugs fit into the toolbox of treatment options. Fingolimod has been shown to be effective in decreasing the risk of relapse, slowing progression of disability, and lessening the chance of new MRI lesions. The drug is taken as a once-daily pill. It's main mechanism of action is to keep certain immune cells from getting into the blood and then into the CNS. Safety issues include the risk of a decreased heart rate after the first dose, infections such as shingles, swelling in a part of the retina called the macula, and pulmonary complications. Although approved as a first-line agent, many neurologists are using it more as a second-line therapy for those who have failed to adequately respond to other DMTs. Since the drug was first introduced, several deaths have been reported in patients who were given Gilenya who had preexisting heart conditions. Now, the preadministration monitoring and first dose monitoring of this drug is stricter, and it is contraindicated for persons with certain types of heart conditions and who are on certain types of heart medications.

A second oral agent, teriflunimide (Aubagio), indicated for the treatment of relapsing forms of MS, was approved by the FDA in October 2012. It is a form of a drug that has been used for the past 10 years to treat rheumatoid arthritis and works by reducing the number of white blood cells. Aubagio is taken once a day. Its side effects include lowered white blood cell count and liver irritation, so people on this drug must have periodic blood tests to monitor these levels. Additionally Aubagio can cause (what is usually) temporary hair loss. Aubagio can cause birth defects and may persist in the body for up to 2 years after treatment is stopped. Thus patients with MS who are considering treatment with Aubagio and who are thinking of starting a family (this includes both men and women) will need to discuss this with their neurologist. A protocol to rapidly eliminate the drug from the system (over about 2 weeks) exists and can be used under the direction of a physician and would be appropriate to use if conception was being considered.

Tecfidera, the newest oral DMT, was FDA approved in April 2013. Its active compound, dimethyl fumarate, has been used in Europe for about 20 years to treat psoriasis. Tecfidera is taken by mouth two times a day after an initial dose titration. It was found through several clinical trials to reduce new inflammation and relapses and to have some effect on progression. It is thought to work partly by shifting an inflammatory immune response to an anti-inflammatory one, and also appears to reduce oxidative stress in the CNS. Its side effects include a flushing sensation and gastrointestinal symptoms such as abdominal pain, nausea, cramping, and diarrhea. These side effects usually go away after the first 2 to 3 months and are lessened by taking the medication with food. Persons who are taking Tecfidera also require blood tests to monitor blood count and liver functions. In 2014, there was a report of the death of an individual who after 3+ years of Tecfidera, developed PML (progressive multifocal leukoencelopathy) a rare and potentially fatal brain infection. This case underscores the need for close follow-up and regular monitoring of blood cell counts. See Table 5–1 for a listing of all the FDA-approved DMTs.

Relapsing-remitting MS can over time transition into secondary-progressive MS. No definitive data shows that treatment with DMTs prevents this transition, but they clearly increase relapse-free time, particularly early on in the disease. In addition, each has demonstrated some positive effect on the delay disability progression. In secondary-progressive MS that with continued relapses, the DMT drugs are likely to be effective. However, when there is progression and no evidence of relapses or new inflammation, the efficacy of the DMTs is less clear.

Reproductive Issues

Women of childbearing age represent a significant portion of the MS community. Therefore, the potential effects of DMTs on fertility, pregnancy, and the developing baby are of great importance. The FDA has a system for characterizing medications based on their potential to produce harm to a developing fetus (see Table 5–2). Beta interferons are categorized as Pregnancy Category C. Registries of women who have become pregnant while on beta interferons have shown a slight increase in the risk of early miscarriage and slightly lower birthweights in the babies. Copaxone is a Pregnancy Category B medication. Human registries have also shown no risk to mother or baby from Copaxone. Tysabri, Gilenya, Tecfidera, and Lemtrada

TABLE 5–2 US Food and Drug Administration Classification of Pregnancy Risk Categories

A	No harm in human studies
B	No known harm in animal studies
C	Known harm in animal or human studies
D	Known harm in humans; use may be justified in pregnancy in some cases
X	Known harm in humans; use not justified

are all Category C drugs; and Novantrone is a Category D drug (see also Chapter 7 on reproductive issues).

Aubagio is a pregnancy Category X drug—its use is associated with known fetal harm and use is contraindicated during pregnancy. Women of childbearing age must have a negative pregnancy text before starting the drug and must use effective birth control while on it. This drug is also Category X for men. Men on Aubagio who father a child have a higher risk of seeing birth defects in that child.

TABLE 5–3 Pregnancy Categories of Disease-Modifying Therapies

Disease-Modifying Therapy	Pregnancy Category
Avonex	C
Betaseron/Extavia	C
Rebif	C
Plegridy	C
Copaxone	B
Novantrone	D
Tysabri	C
Gilenya	C
Aubagio	X
Fingolimod	C
Lemtrada	C

Table 5–3 lists the pregnancy categories for each FDA approved DMT.

Which Disease-Modifying Therapy Is the Best?

There is no one "best" DMT that is right for everyone. The various drugs all have different mechanisms of action and different degrees of efficacy in reduction of relapses as well as more- or less-severe side effect profiles. Because very few head-to-head trials have been conducted between the different DMTs, it cannot definitively be stated that one drug is more effective than another. The effects of each DMT tested against a placebo (inactive compound) are shown in Table 5–4. Which DMT is recommended for a specific patient depends on many factors, including disease activity, presence of other medical conditions, and lifestyle issues such as career and

TABLE 5–4 Effectiveness of US Food and Drug Administration–Approved Disease-Modifying Therapies Compared to Placebo

Medication	Reduction in Relapses (Compared to Placebo)	Reduction in Inflammation on MRI (Compared to Placebo)
Betaseron/Extavia	34%	80%
Avonex	18%	42%
Rebif	32%	88%
Plegridy	36%	86%
Copaxone	29%	33%
Tysabri	68%	92%
Novantrone	66%	79%
Gilenya	54%	82%
Aubagio	31%	23%–51%
Tecfidera	50%	90%
*Lemtrada	49%	44%

*Lemtrada was compared to beta interferon, not a placebo.

family. It is not uncommon to switch medications because of lack of efficacy or intolerability. The best DMT is the one that is right for your particular case.

Summary

The ability to modify the MS disease process through drug therapies represents a significant leap in our understanding of this disease. Medications currently available offer the possibility of decreasing the frequency of relapses, slowing the progression of disability, and lessening the likelihood of new lesions. It is hoped that further research will lead to the emergence of options that are even more convenient and effective. Clinical trials of new drugs may yet yield new medications for modifying the secondary-progressive and primary-progressive courses of the disease.

Chapter 6

Lifestyle Management

In this chapter you'll learn:

- **How to deal with fatigue**
- **How multiple sclerosis affects mood**
- **The specific benefits of exercise for persons with multiple sclerosis**
- **Wellness strategies important for persons with multiple sclerosis**

Multiple sclerosis (MS) is an insidious disease. Its symptoms can creep into many aspects of a person's daily life, making everything from brushing hair to driving a car to buying groceries more difficult. In addition to attempting to slow the course of the disease itself, people with MS also must find ways to manage its many and varied symptoms so that they can still live the lives that they want.

This chapter addresses the ways in which many of the most common MS symptoms can interfere with a person's regular daily activities and explains strategies for lessening their impact.

Finding Relief from Multiple Sclerosis–Related Fatigue

From time to time, everybody experiences fatigue—that weariness and sense of exhaustion that comes from certain kinds of exertion, labor, or stress. The difference between everyday fatigue and

MS-related fatigue is that the latter can consistently interfere with an individual's ability to carry out his or her usual activities.

Fatigue is not only the most common symptom among people with MS, but it is also the one that many describe as the most bothersome. Indeed, it is one of the two main reasons why some who have MS leave the workforce. (The other is cognitive dysfunction, or the impairment of thinking, which is discussed later in this chapter as well as in Chapter 4.)

People with MS describe their fatigue with expressions such as, "It's like swimming with a fur coat on," and, "I feel like I'm lying down with a lead blanket over me." The imagery is vivid—but in reality, fatigue is invisible. You can't look at a person with MS and assess his or her fatigue level. Friends and family may not understand why those experiencing MS fatigue can no longer do all the things they once did. And coworkers or supervisors may conclude that the person is simply lazy or unmotivated. Multiple sclerosis–related fatigue thus contributes to difficulties both at home and at work.

Sharon has relapsing-remitting MS. Her MS was diagnosed 3 years ago, when she was 34 years old. She has had two relapses but has recovered well from them. Friends and family tell her frequently, "You look great. I can't believe you have MS." Some days, Sharon doesn't feel great. In spite of getting good sleep, she sometimes experiences severe fatigue. "It seems to come from nowhere," Sharon explains. "I'll get this overwhelming wave of tiredness. It's like I weigh a thousand pounds and just can't do any more. My husband tries to understand, but I know it frustrates him too. I sometimes wonder if he thinks I'm just lazy." Sharon discusses

(Continued)

(Continued)
her fatigue with her neurologist, and, together, they review lifestyle changes and possible medical treatments for MS-related fatigue along with other factors that can contribute to improving her fatigue, such as regular exercise.

Defining Primary and Secondary Multiple Sclerosis Fatigue

There are two basic types of MS-related fatigue. The first, **primary MS fatigue**, is largely a symptom of the disease itself. The other, **secondary MS fatigue**, is due to other factors that come into play once the disease is underway, such as sleep disruption, side effects from medication, and the increased effort required to perform daily activities. Secondary factors often make primary MS fatigue worse. Also, other illness, such as anemia, low-thyroid function, and infections, may produce fatigue that can be confused with MS fatigue.

Relieving Primary Fatigue with Exercise

Primary MS fatigue is divided into two subtypes: **lassitude** and **nerve fiber fatigue**. Lassitude is an overwhelming sense of tiredness that materializes out of the blue. It is not necessarily associated with exertion or heat exposure, but in some instances it can be exacerbated by factors such as heat, stress, sleep disruption, or medications.

One way for people with MS to relieve lassitude is with regular exercise. Exercise may include some combination of aerobic, resistance, and stretching routines. On the surface, it might sound counterintuitive to tell a fatigued person to exercise. In fact, it was not long ago that people with MS were pointedly told not to exercise for fear they might use up what little energy they had. Skier

Jimmie Heuga won the Olympic bronze medal in 1964 and was diagnosed with MS in 1970. His biography sums up the medical community's thoughts on MS and exercise at that time: "When Jimmie was diagnosed with MS, doctors advised him to avoid physical activity because it was thought that it would exacerbate his symptoms."

In contrast to these long-held assumptions, a significant body of research has shown that, in general, people with MS not only tolerate exercise well but also find that it improves the quality of their lives. Surprisingly, even those with more advanced disability can benefit from exercise, although the type of exercise that is possible will vary based on the level of disability. Among the benefits of exercise for people with MS are improved physical strength, muscle tone, balance, and coordination, as well as aid in counteracting depression. By contrast, not exercising can lead a person with MS-related lassitude into a spiral of increased fatigue, deconditioning, and depression.

Exercise has not generally been found to help with the second type of primary MS fatigue, nerve fiber fatigue. About 70% of people with MS may experience some form of nerve fiber fatigue due to their MS. This means that with heat exposure or exertion, they may experience a temporary worsening of a neurologic symptom. It's important to note that these temporary symptoms are not relapses and are not an indication of new damage or harm for the person with MS. The person with MS may find that these symptoms come on with only a few minutes of exercise one day and not at all during another exercise session. Cooling strategies are often helpful in improving this kind of fatigue.

In general, when an exercise brings on worsening of a neurologic symptom, it may be wise to rest and cool off until the symptom resolves. A recurring theme you'll hear when thinking about exercise in MS is flexibility. The trick is to find an exercise program that works for you. That may mean finding exercises that are less likely to provoke temporary worsening of neurologic symptoms.

There is no single "best" kind of exercise program for people with MS. Effective programs might, for instance, involve a combination of light weights, stretching, walking, yoga, aquatics, biking, and so on. Factors influencing which approach suits the individual include the availability of resources and transportation, the person's level of ability, and his or her relative sensitivity to heat and exertion. For example, swimming can be a good choice for those with MS who are sensitive to heat. Exercise options for people with MS will be discussed in detail later on in this chapter.

Relieving Lassitude with Medications

When exercise proves to be inadequate, medications can be used to help relieve primary MS fatigue. Amantidine (Symmetrel) is a drug that, when introduced in 1964, was used to stave off influenza. Unexpectedly, it was also found to boost energy levels in some people with MS. When amantidine is taken twice daily, about half of those with the disease find it helpful in reducing fatigue. Generally, a person can recognize whether this drug is working after using it for 2 to 4 weeks. Some find that the effectiveness of amantidine decreases over time. However, taking a several-day break from the drug and then resuming use may enable it to work effectively again. Generally, the risk of side effects with amantidine is low. If taken too late in the day, it can cause insomnia.

Modafinil (Provigil) is a prescription drug that promotes wakefulness and alertness. It was originally developed to treat another neurologic disorder, narcolepsy, which is characterized by abnormal and sudden sleepiness. It has also been studied by the military as an alternative to amphetamines in situations where troops face lengthy periods of sleep deprivation and must remain alert.

Several studies examining modafinil's effectiveness for MS-related lassitude have shown that it provides some benefit. Modafinil is generally taken once or twice daily, but some people report it to be beneficial when used only on an as-needed basis. It should not be taken too late in the day because it may cause sleep problems. The risk of side effects is low, but occasionally modafinil can produce jitteriness. In addition some people experience othereside effects such as headache, nausea, and rapid heart rate. Insurance coverage for modafinil use in MS can sometimes be a problem because of the high cost of the drug and the fact that it is not approved by the US Food and Drug Administration (FDA) for MS-related fatigue. A newer form of the drug, called armodafanil (Nuvigil), was approved by the FDA in 2007 for the treatment of excessive sleepiness associated with narcolepsy, obstructive sleep apnea, and shift work sleep disorder. This form allows for once-daily dosing but otherwise has the same benefits and potential side effects as modafinil.

Before modafinil became available, various prescription stimulants were commonly used to counteract MS-related fatigue, including methylphenidate (Ritalin) and the mixture of amphetamine and dextroamphetamine (Adderall). Although both carry the potential for tolerance or addiction, experience shows that this generally does not become a major problem. A 2009 study by the National Institute on Drug Abuse found a low potential for tolerance or addiction when Ritalin was used for medical purposes. Since these stimulants are classed as controlled substances, prescriptions must be renewed by the physician rather than refilled at the patient's request.

Antidepressant medications may be helpful as well—particularly, of course, when fatigue is associated with depression. Some MS symptoms seem to play off one another. Specifically, it is not unusual to see fatigue, depression, and cognitive problems all operating in the same person. Distinguishing between MS-related fatigue and depression-related fatigue can be tricky. People with MS fatigue want to participate in an activity, but their bodies resist going along for the ride. In depression-related fatigue, the desire to participate in activities may be greatly reduced. Fatigue from either source will generally diminish the ability to concentrate, which tends to make cognitive problems seem worse. Since people with MS can have some or all of these problems from time to time, antidepressants may serve to increase energy and improve both mood and concentration. It should be noted that the use of all of these medications for MS fatigue is considered off label as they are not FDA approved for this indication.

Nerve Fiber Fatigue

This subtype of primary MS fatigue is a direct byproduct of demyelination, which, as earlier chapters have explained, is damage to myelin—the fatty insulation that protects nerve fibers (axons) and helps them transmit signals from the central nervous system to the rest of the body. Once a nerve fiber has been demyelinated, it can still send signals, but not as well as a normally myelinated (insulated) axon can. Thus, demyelinated axons are weak links in the impulse-transmission chain. When these damaged nerve fibers are overused or become overheated, such as during sustained exertion or when body temperature rises, the nerves involved become less and less able to send signals. This is called conduction block. Conduction block is not permanent; once the body rests and cools off, the nerve fibers start working again.

Joseph, who has MS, goes out for a walk. After a couple of blocks, he notices his foot dragging a little. After another few blocks, this dragging grows more pronounced. He returns home, and after a few hours everything is back to normal. If it happens to be very hot outside, the weakness may occur with even less exertion. While this may seem to contradict the advice to get exercise presented in this chapter, it's important to know not only that neurologic symptoms worsened by exertion or heat are temporary but also that

(Continued)

(Continued)

they can be readily managed and prevented. In this case, the heat-related foot weakness might have responded to Joseph cooling himself off with an icy drink, a cold towel, or splashing cold water on his hands and face.

It is interesting to note that some people with MS are not at all bothered by heat or exertion. And some actually have problems when their bodies get too cold—usually, a worsening of muscle spasticity. So it's important to remember that your symptoms are unique to you, and it's important to discuss them with your doctor so that both of you are informed and so that you can live a long and productive life.

Anything done to lower the body temperature will delay or even prevent the occurrence of nerve fiber fatigue symptoms brought on by heat exposure or exertion. Cooling vests, for example, can help a person with MS function better in hot conditions. Certain kinds of cooling neck wraps and hats also help keep the body cool, as do cold beverages.

Secondary Multiple Sclerosis Fatigue

As noted, secondary MS fatigue can be caused by several factors, such as sleep disruption, response to medications, or other medical conditions that can produce fatigue, none of which are directly due to MS.

Unfortunately, some medications used for managing MS can actually cause drowsiness or fatigue. Among these are antidepressants, medications used to treat spasticity, and many pain medications. With certain of these medications, a reduction in energy levels may be temporary. For example, some people starting one of the beta interferon therapies described in Chapter 5 may experience fatigue while their bodies adjust to the medication.

When arm or leg muscles grow weak or tire quickly due to MS, it becomes more difficult to perform normal daily activities. This extra exertion leads to more fatigue. Some people experience a roller-coaster pattern of fluctuating energy levels. In this regard, physical and occupational therapy, in which individuals learn how to work smarter rather than harder, can help. By planning activities in ways that conserve energy, it may be possible to pace oneself and attain more consistent energy levels.

Jim, aged 54, has secondary-progressive MS. He has always been a hard worker. According to his wife: "Jim comes in two speeds, asleep and 100 miles per hour. Some days, he wakes up feeling pretty energetic. On those days, he tries to cram 3 days' worth of work into 1 day. I've tried to get him to pace himself, but he says he wants to get as much done as possible since he doesn't know if he'll feel this good tomorrow." Jim admits that when he does this, the "good" day is typically followed by several days of poor energy and a decreased ability to get much done. After describing this pattern to his neurologist, Jim is referred to an occupational therapist to work on energy conservation. Jim says, "I really didn't want to go to see the therapist, but after some gentle coaxing from my wife, I did. I have to admit, some of the advice from the therapist has helped me pace myself. I now have fewer days when I'm really wiped out."

Other Contributors to Fatigue and Sleep Disorders

People with MS can also have other medical conditions that cause fatigue, such as anemia or low thyroid levels, and these conditions can combine with MS symptoms to further drag a person down.

Often doctors will check to see whether these conditions are present in persons with MS who report fatigue. Other medical conditions that can aggravate MS fatigue are sleep disorders such as sleep apnea or **restless legs syndrome.**

Sleep disruption can contribute to low daytime energy. Sleep may be interrupted by muscle spasms, the need to empty the bladder at night, or loss of bladder control. Depression can also interfere with getting a good night's sleep. Treatments that reduce these symptoms will also likely reduce sleep disruption–related fatigue. (Treatments for spasticity and bladder problems are discussed in Chapter 4.) Other sleep disorders, such as restless legs syndrome, are actually more common in persons with MS and require specific treatment. When a primary sleep disorder is suspected, referral to a physician who specializes in sleep medicine is often very helpful for proper diagnosis and treatment.

Sometimes a specific cause of sleep disruption cannot be pinned down. Some people just have a hard time getting to sleep, staying asleep, or both. Seeing a doctor to discuss sleep hygiene—a fancy term for maintaining good sleep habits—as well as the risks and benefits of medications that facilitate sleep, is recommended.

Summary

Fatigue is a challenge for many people with MS. Lassitude and nerve fiber fatigue are due to MS itself, but various non-MS-related factors also come into play. Careful assessment of the symptoms is needed to determine the cause of the fatigue so that the most appropriate and useful treatment plan can be developed. As with most symptoms of MS, approaching fatigue management from different angles is most useful—so combining of the use of medication, rehabilitation strategies to increase activity level, and lifestyle modifications that maximize available energy and reduce energy waste are likely to be most helpful.

How Multiple Sclerosis Affects Mood

As detailed in preceding chapters, MS is a complex disease in which the nerves of the brain and spinal cord are attacked and damaged by the body's own immune system. Because of this, the central nervous system's ability to send and receive nerve signals is disrupted, and one or more of various symptoms—involving mobility, eyesight, sensation, waste elimination, mental processing, and mood—can, depending on the degree of damage, result. The symptoms, including mood, vary considerably among individuals, both in type and intensity. Mood is defined as the state of one's emotions. Of course, everybody experiences and displays various emotions at different times. In most cases, mood changes are temporary and do not have a serious impact on how a person functions. Some people, however, experience unsettling or low moods or a series of mood fluctuations that interfere with their daily lives to the extent that it becomes a medical problem. Mood disorder is a psychiatric term for classifying mood problems; mood disorders are generally categorized either as mostly depressed or as overly elevated (manic).

Multiple sclerosis can have both an immediate and a long-term impact on one's emotions. Depression is associated with many chronic illnesses and is the most common mood disorder associated with MS. Estimates are that about 50% of people with MS will need to cope with clinical or major depression at some point in their lifetime. Even more troubling is that suicide is more common in people with MS than in those dealing with other chronic illnesses.

These are surely difficult and worrying statistics to read. Fortunately, many effective treatments for mood disorders exist that can help to manage these difficult symptoms. We'll talk more about these options after exploring depression and other mood changes that can be involved with MS in more detail.

Adjustment-Related Mood Disorder

A number of factors can underlie depression associated with MS.

Individuals often react to learning they have MS with denial, disbelief, anger, fear, or depression. This can prompt a reactive depression—also known as an adjustment-related disorder with depressed mood.

Multiple sclerosis is also very unpredictable and, while the way it progresses can vary widely among people with the disorder, it is very likely to cause unwanted lifestyle changes at some point during its course. These changes, the unpredictability of the changes, and the difficulty of adapting to and coping with symptoms—an ongoing process—may provoke feelings of depression at different times.

Depression can also be caused by inflammation and demyelination that occurs within the central nervous system. Advanced imaging studies have suggested that abnormalities in certain brain regions are associated with symptoms of depression. Mood can also be negatively altered by some medications.

As noted in Chapter 3, the process of diagnosing MS can take a long time. Many individuals are sure that *something* is wrong, but often the symptoms are vague, and it can require months and even years of testing before MS is finally diagnosed (or ruled out). Finally learning that MS is the source of the trouble can be, in some sense, a relief—at last you know what's wrong! This emotion is often quickly replaced with uneasiness about what the future may hold, an uneasiness that starts with questions such as these: Should I tell my family? My employer? Can I date? Should I get married? Should I apply for a new job? Can I have children? Will I end up in a wheelchair? Will I become a burden to my family? These questions are nearly impossible to answer with complete accuracy, particularly soon after diagnosis. Worry and concern about the future can prompt feelings of sadness and depression.

Someone who has just been diagnosed with MS commonly experiences not only fear, but feelings of sadness and anger about what might happen next. In any of those mental states, it may seem impossible to make decisions about the future. This type of depressed emotion can recur as new symptoms emerge or if a particular physical ability becomes more impaired due to an ongoing MS symptom. New questions arise—such as, Will I be able to walk again? Will my vision get better? Will my energy return? The symptoms, and the returning feelings of uncertainty, can make one's mood change again—and a new adjustment may need to take place.

People going through an adjustment-related mood disorder as a result of an MS diagnosis also may experience symptoms such as irritability, fatigue, trouble sleeping, changes in appetite, withdrawal, trouble concentrating, and loss of interest in normally pleasurable activities. Not infrequently, individuals may have feelings of hopelessness that can be overwhelming.

These are important symptoms to share with your neurologist and your primary care doctor. Mood disorders are treatable. Counseling or psychotherapy as well as medications may be needed to treat a mood disorder.

While some individuals are reluctant to take medications for mood disorders or to enter into counseling or psychotherapy, it is important to realize that symptoms of a mood disorder should be as aggressively treated as any physical symptom of MS. It is vital for individuals with MS to keep their doctors up-to-date about their emotional state.

Medications for Depression and Mood Disorders

Various prescription medications are available to treat depression and have been shown to be highly effective for many individuals. These medications affect brain chemicals that are associated with mood and are classified according to the specific chemicals they influence. Antidepressants are categorized as follows:

1. **Tricyclic antidepressants.** Tricyclic antidepressants such as amitriptyline (Elavil) or nortryptyline (Pamelor) have been used for many years to treat depression. Although they are effective, they tend to be sedating and overall have more side effects associated with them than do the other classes of antidepressants listed below. Side effects common with tricyclics are drowsiness, dry mouth, blurred vision, constipation, low sex drive, rapid heart rate, and increased appetite.

2. **Selective serotonin reuptake inhibitors.** Selective serotonin reuptake inhibitors (SSRIs) are newer and tend to have fewer and different side effects then the tricyclic antidepressants. These drugs primarily have an effect on the brain chemical serotonin. Possible side effects may include nausea, change in weight, drowsiness, headache, dizziness, and impaired sexual function. Some of the SSRIs are:
   - Fluoxetine (Prozac)
   - Sertraline (Zoloft)
   - Paroxetine (Paxil)
   - Citalopram (Celexa)
   - Escitalopram (Lexapro)

3. **Serotonin-norepinephrine reuptake inhibitors.** Serotonin-norepinephrine reuptake inhibitors (SNRIs) have an effect on two brain chemicals, serotonin and norepinephrine, and can be helpful to some people. One of them, duloxetine, is also used to treat certain types of nerve-related pain, such as the pain experienced with fibromyalgia or the pain in the extremities sometimes associated with diabetes. Side effects possible with SNRIs include drowsiness, dizziness, fatigue, headache, mydriasis (dilated pupils),

nausea/vomiting, sexual dysfunction, change in weight, and urinary retention. SNRIs include:
- Venlafaxine (Effexor)
- Duloxetine (Cymbalta)
- Desvenlafaxine (Pristiq)

4. **Unique Antidepressant.** Bupropion (Wellbutrin, Zyban) is considered a unique antidepressant. Bupropion tends to be more energizing than other antidepressants. It does not cause weight gain or sexual side effects as can other antidepressants; on the other hand, it can cause headaches and can also provoke seizures, particularly in high doses.

The effectiveness of any of these antidepressants varies depending on the individual. You may have to try more than one of them before finding the medication that works most effectively and has the fewest undesirable side effects. Each of the antidepressants has possible side effects, and individual responses to the drugs will vary. It is very important to work closely with your prescribing physician to determine the most effective and best-tolerated medication. It is also very important to discuss any change in the dose with your physician and to never abruptly stop the medication, as a withdrawal syndrome may occur.

Many people who experience a change in their mood after the diagnosis of MS want to know if the mood change is due to their reaction to the disease or to the disease itself. While this determination is not easily made, it is important to know that the treatment is the same. Counseling, as well as medication, is used to optimally treat symptoms of depression.

Other Disturbances of Mood

Although depression is the most common mood disorder seen in MS, other mood disorders can occur. For example, some people with the disease find themselves laughing or crying uncontrollably or disproportionately to whatever is happening at the moment, even if what is happening is not particularly funny or sad. These episodes are unpredictable and occur as "outbursts," not connected to any particular event. These inappropriate emotions are caused by nerve damage in a specific part of the brain, that is, they are a result of the MS. The medical term for this symptom is pseudobulbar affect (PBA). Naturally, they can be upsetting to the individual and to those present. It is important that everybody involved understands the source of such outbursts as well as that they are beyond the individual's control. Occasionally, the doctor may try a type of antidepressant medication to help lessen these kinds of emotional outbursts. A new medication Nuedexta, which is a combination of two older medications, was approved to specifically treat this symptom. Tricyclic antidepressants are also sometimes useful in treating this problem.

A less common form of mood change is euphoria, in which the individual is happy or elated out of proportion with expectations or in relation to the given situation. Often, MS-related euphoria leads individuals to brush off or laugh off changes in their symptoms or physical abilities. Usually, euphoria is associated with changes in mental ability, such as memory loss or other impaired cognitive abilities.

Summary

About 50% of people who are newly diagnosed with MS experience mood difficulties; these usually take the form of depression. Yet it is important to know that once the emotional reaction to the diagnosis has been absorbed, most people build a positive sense of themselves and find proactive ways to cope with the condition. Individuals who become depressed can be treated effectively, so long as they and their doctors maintain open and honest communication. Once treatment has begun, it is important to stick with it, since depression takes time to subside. If antidepressant drugs are part of the treatment, they should not be stopped abruptly. Doctors should be informed of every medication you are taking, including over-the-counter drugs and herbal remedies, as these can interact with other medications and have harmful side effects.

Exercise and Multiple Sclerosis

The word *exercise* brings different images to mind for each person. For many, the word creates an overall image of physical fitness. Some people picture weightlifters, while others visualize runners or cyclists and still others visualize an aerobics class. In addition, most people believe that exercise involves putting great stress on the body—the "no pain, no gain" philosophy. Given all that, many people with MS cannot picture themselves exercising routinely and don't believe they have the strength or endurance for it. They may even have heard that exercise is harmful to those with the disease; however, multiple research studies describing the outcomes of exercise in MS patients describe benefits of exercise. Patients who exercise have experienced improved strength and endurance, reduced fatigue, and improved mood.

Exercise has shown benefit both in patients mildly affected by MS and in those with more physical impairment. Numerous studies using various exercise regimens have reported positive effects of exercise on such MS symptoms as fatigue, weakness, and depression and improved quality of life.

As noted earlier, fatigue is the most typical complaint among people with MS. Many have enough energy to go to work but have little or none left over at the end of the day for physical activities such as exercise. In addition, exercise usually raises the body's temperature, and heat sensitivity is common in MS. While increased body heat and exposure to external heat do not themselves worsen the disease, they can temporarily cause symptoms to flare up. Often, exposure to heat increases fatigue and makes a person with MS feel weak. For these reasons, avoidance of regular exercise becomes the norm for many people with MS.

The basic health benefits of routine exercise for most people are well-known. Exercise can:

- Help elevate mood as well as reduce stress and anxiety
- Lessen the impact of chronic conditions such as osteoporosis, high blood pressure, high blood sugar, and high cholesterol
- Help in weight loss and weight management
- Improve cardiac function, stamina, and endurance
- Counteract fatigue

People with MS can attain many of the same benefits from exercise as other people do. In fact, research on the effects of regular exercise among people with the disorder has shown improvements in cardiovascular health, strength, and stamina. In addition, exercise has been found to improve their bowel and bladder function as well as raise their mood. Most importantly, numerous studies indicate that there is no evidence that exercise harms individuals with MS.

Given that effects of MS on individuals vary widely, the question becomes, how does someone create an aerobic exercise program that is right for his or her particular needs?

The National MS Society recommends that exercise programs for people with MS should be individually designed by rehabilitation specialists who are familiar with and knowledgeable about MS.

When planning an exercise regimen, a person with MS and the rehabilitation specialist should consider the following:

- Purpose of exercise (aerobic, strength, balance, coordination)
- Duration (how long to exercise at each session)
- Frequency (how many times per day or week to exercise)
- Intensity (how vigorous the exercise should be)

Since everyone experiences MS differently and has different levels of physical ability, there can be no "cookbook" approach to developing an exercise plan. In addition, the nature of whatever exercise regimen a person may have followed before being diagnosed will have an impact on whatever post-diagnosis plan is decided on. For instance, a person who has never exercised regularly prior to the MS diagnosis may have difficulty adhering to an exercise program. In contrast, a person who exercised vigorously prior to the MS diagnosis may try to overexercise or be disappointed if he or she cannot exercise at the same level as before developing MS. As part of shaping the overall plan, a physical therapist can identify problem areas and target them with the appropriate exercises. Certain kinds of exercise have been found to be particularly beneficial in MS. For example, yoga is helpful in decreasing spasticity and increasing the mobility of joints in the legs, arms, hands, and feet. It has also been found in some studies to lessen fatigue and increase strength. Aquatherapy—exercises done in a pool—can help as well. The buoyancy of the water provides support and puts less strain on joints, and the water can be used as resistance that strengthens muscles. A pool temperature between 80°F and 85°F will keep the body temperature from becoming elevated.

Many people are able to continue their prediagnosis exercise regimen without any restrictions or modifications. However, the plan needs to be specifically tailored in cases where symptoms such as fatigue, heat intolerance, imbalance, weakness, or spasticity are present. It is vital to be aware that the "no pain, no gain" approach is inappropriate in MS—and also unnecessary in order to produce improvement. Additionally, it is not helpful—indeed, it is counterproductive—to exercise until one is overheated.

The long-term success of any MS-oriented exercise plan—indeed, of exercise in general—is rooted in persistence; it will work only if the individual sticks with it.

People with MS who exercise should:

- Be evaluated by their primary care physicians prior to initiating or resuming an exercise program
- Discuss exercise with their MS specialist

- Develop an individualized exercise plan in collaboration with an MS rehabilitation specialist
- Warm up muscles with stretching
- Perform exercises slowly
- Rest frequently and avoid exercising to the point of exhaustion
- Keep body temperature down with cool beverages or cooling garments, such as a cooling vest or collar
- Wear lightweight clothing
- If using a pool, be sure the water temperature is between 80°F and 85°F

Exercise plans can be specifically fashioned to deal with symptoms commonly experienced in MS.

Physical Therapy

In addition to physical activities such as aerobic or resistance activities described above, physical therapy, which is targeted structured exercises and strategies designed to help over come a specific deficit such as weakness, is very valuable to helping to improve or maintain function in persons with MS. A physical therapist may recommend exercises for MS symptoms such as weakness, spasticity, discomfort, imbalance, and reduced stamina. Some plans may call for the use of an assistive device, such as a cane or a crutch. Although many people resist the idea of using these devices, they often can help counteract fatigue, alleviate discomfort, and steady the gait.

> Steve, who was diagnosed with MS when he was 36, noticed he was tripping over his right toe several times each day. While 6 months ago he could walk 10 blocks or more without
>
> *(Continued)*

(Continued)

rest, he reached a point where he could walk only about three blocks before he felt stiffness and weakness in his right leg and an overall sense of exhaustion. Steve had never exercised on a regular basis prior to being diagnosed, and he was convinced that his fatigue prevented him from doing so now. His doctor referred him to a physical therapist who had a working familiarity with MS. The therapist prescribed a program that included exercises to strengthen Steve's hip, buttocks, and trunk muscles, plus stretching exercises to address his tight calf muscles. These exercises were fitted into his workday and proved not to be taxing. After about 6 weeks, Steve's walking improved, and he tripped less often.

Regular exercise to achieve—or maintain—overall fitness is important for people who have MS and should be made part of an individual's plan for managing the disease. The exercise routine may need to be modified because of specific limitations and symptoms. In addition, exercise plans can be adapted in order to lessen certain symptoms.

How to Work for Wellness with Multiple Sclerosis

"Wellness" is a buzzword heard often in the media and in the healthcare arena. But what does it mean—both generally and specifically in relation to MS? After a person has been diagnosed with MS, his or her primary focus quite naturally is on the disease itself—recognizing and dealing with its symptoms and seeking appropriate medical treatments and physical therapies. This focus can leave little room to consider the rest of one's self. Yet as difficult as it may seem at first, it is important to see MS as an illness that is part of one's life and not as an enveloping new self-definition. Indeed it is feasible, not to mention desirable, to pursue wellness while dealing with this chronic disease.

People have customarily believed that to be considered "well," they must, simply put, not be ill. However, in recent times wellness has come to be understood more broadly—that is, to be viewed on a continuum and on an individual basis. Thus wellness is now seen as the ongoing process through which each person finds ways to achieve a healthy balance among mind, body, and spirit that produces a sense of well-being. Wellness is a multidimensional state of being—attained and maintained in each individual.

Working toward this state of being requires active participation in wellness-focused activities. The benefits of exercise and the recognition and treatment of mood disorders have already been discussed in this chapter. Additional areas for pursuing wellness include nutrition, preventive healthcare, stress management, personal relationship health, and spiritual health.

Nutrition

Much has been written about nutrition with regard to MS, with an emphasis on dietary adjustments. A quick Google search using the keywords "diet and MS" yields about 74 million pages! A slightly refined search, using "MS diet," provides nearly 72 million pages. Clearly, this is a topic of great interest! Unfortunately, of course, just about anybody can create a website and make claims about anything. So how, amid this flood of data, can you find information that is actually worthwhile and discern which MS-oriented diets are generally beneficial?

Diet has been studied as a possible risk factor in the development of MS, and epidemiologic population studies have suggested that those with diets high in animal fat have an increased risk for

MS. However, other studies that have been done to attempt to prove this suggestion have not had consistent results, so the idea that MS is caused by diets high in animal fat has not been proven.

To date no specific diet has been proven to reduce the risk of developing MS or found to have any effect on symptoms, relapses, or progression of the disease. Despite the lack of proof, one can still find MS diets on the Internet and in books. Two diets that have received particular attention are the Swank Diet and the Weil MS Diet.

The Swank Diet has received considerable publicity in the MS community. Dr. Roy Swank was a neurologist and head of the department of neurology at Oregon Health and Science University for 22 years. He believed that dietary modification would help lessen or modify the MS disease process as well as the symptoms of the disease. The Swank diet is very low in saturated (animal) fats and unsaturated fats, red meat, dairy fat, and processed foods. Dr. Swank studied 144 people with MS for over 30 years. He reported in 1990 that those who had followed his diet had a less severe course of MS then those who did not follow the diet. The results of his research have been questioned and criticized for certain flaws in the way the study was conducted. For example, there was no control group who did not follow the diet, so it is not known if the improvements would have occurred anyway, as sometimes happens in persons with MS. Thus, without evidence from a well-designed, controlled clinical trial or trials, the Swank diet is not considered a therapeutic approach to the treatment of MS.

Dr. Andrew Weil is a well-known author who is a proponent of integrative medicine. He believes that alternative types of interventions, particularly diet modifications, exercise, and stress management strategies, should always be a part of medical recommendations. He believes that plant-based medications or herbal medicines should be complementary to conventional medicine. He has published many books on healthy living and diet and has made recommendations for a diet for people with MS. Dr. Weil's diet recommends reduction in animal proteins, elimination of milk products, elimination of trans fats (fats made in the laboratory to preserve the shelf life of foods), and any partially hydrogenated fats. In addition he recommends foods high in omega-3 fatty acids. This diet does bear some similarity to Dr. Swank's diet, but no controlled trials have been conducted to prove the claims of benefit in MS. Additionally, lean meat and dairy products contain several important nutrients, including certain vitamins and minerals such as calcium and iron that are important for good health, so such a diet is not only of no proven benefit but could potentially produce poor nutrition.

Most recently Dr. Terry Wahls, who has MS, has published her thoughts on MS treatment, which includes the Wahls Paleo Diet as well as other interventions. The Paleo Diet is based on that of hunter-gatherer ancestors and includes foods that are high in protein, such as meats and seafood, low in sugar and glycemic index, moderately high in healthy oils (e.g., olive, flaxseed, walnut), and high in fresh fruits and vegetables. What is noticeably absent from this type of diet is cereal grains, processed foods, sugar, and salt. Both the Paleo Diet and the Wahls Protocol, which is similar, have not been proven to positively impact MS at this time. While Dr. Wahls has stated benefit she derived from her protocol, more research would be necessary to demonstrate efficacy for the majority of people with MS.

Thus to date there is no single proven MS diet. Diet recommendations are therefore for general health and not specific to MS. Generally, a "healthy diet" means eating a wide variety of foods and exercising moderation when it comes to saturated fats, sodium, and sugars.

The US Department of Agriculture's "food pyramid," which everyone learns about in school and which has been updated over the years to reflect advances in research, continues to be a key guide to healthy eating.

Vitamin D

While no specific diet is proven to affect MS risk or disease course, vitamin D has received a good deal of attention because of its importance to the immune system and to bone health. This fat-soluble nutrient is necessary for the body's absorption of calcium. Vitamin D also plays a role in inflammation. Studies in the animal model of MS, known as experimental allergic encephalomyelitis (EAE), demonstrated that vitamin D prevented the development of EAE and lessoned the severity of EAE in previously affected animals. In the EAE model, vitamin D induced anti-inflammatory cytokines, thus reducing the inflammation associated with EAE.

Vitamin D may also play a role in the geographic distribution of MS. Multiple sclerosis is more prevalent the farther one lives from the equator. It is also known that there is less intense sunlight the farther one is from the equator. The major source of vitamin D is from exposure to sunlight. Numerous MS researchers have proposed a role of vitamin D in MS inflammation based on the geographical distribution of the disease and the effects of vitamin D in the animal model of MS, EAE. Epidemiologic studies have shown that subsequent risk of developing MS may be influenced by low vitamin D levels earlier in life. Other research has correlated lower vitamin D levels with increased risk of relapses in persons who already have the disease. If vitamin D is important in the prevention of EAE and may have a role in the development of MS in humans, how much vitamin D does one need to prevent MS or to reduce its severity if MS has already been diagnosed? This is a question that currently has no specific answer. The optimal daily dose of vitamin D and the optimal level of vitamin D in the blood are currently under study. The normal range for total vitamin D varies among laboratories, but is generally 30 mg/mL to 100 mg/mL.

In addition to playing a potential role in preventing MS or reducing inflammation in diagnosed MS, vitamin D is essential for the absorption of calcium. Calcium is vital to bone health. People with MS run a higher risk of developing osteoporosis (thin bones, with less mineral density and more likely to fracture). This is due to less weight bearing if walking or standing is affected by MS, and the use of glucocorticoids (e.g., methylprednisolone, prednisone, dexamethasone), which reduce bone mineralization. Recommended calcium intake for adults ranges from 1,000 to 1,300 mg per day depending on age and gender. Calcium is found in dairy products and in dietary supplements, such as calcium carbonate and calcium citrate. Many calcium supplements contain vitamin D, as well. Recommended vitamin D supplementation for bone health is 800 IU to 1000 IU per day. Persons taking vitamin D supplements should have their vitamin D levels in the blood monitored by a physician, as too much vitamin D can be harmful. It is important to discuss with your physician any supplements that you may be taking, particularly ones such as vitamin D, which need to be monitored.

Other Vitamins

A possible association between vitamin B_{12} and MS has been studied for the past 50 years or more. Vitamin B_{12} is necessary for the body to make myelin. Low or low-normal Vitamin B_{12} blood levels are not uncommon in individuals with MS. Unfortunately, no large studies of vitamin B_{12} in MS have been conducted, and the smaller studies that have been done have shown no conclusive evidence that vitamin B_{12} is a benefit to MS symptoms or to disease management. However, Vitamin B_{12} deficiency can cause neurologic symptoms, such as numbness and tingling in the extremities, difficulty walking, memory loss, and dementia. Vitamin B_{12} levels should be checked, and low levels should be treated with vitamin B_{12} supplementation. Vegetarians should be particularly careful about getting appropriate vitamin B_{12} supplementation, as the primary dietary source of vitamin B_{12} is red meat.

While multivitamin supplementation is not believed to be harmful in MS, no evidence exists at this time to suggest a benefit to multivitamin use, as there are no data that indicate that MS results from a vitamin deficiency, other than the vitamin D data. Some Internet sites suggest antioxidant treatment could be helpful in MS. Again, no evidence exists to support such claims. Treatment with vitamin E and vitamin C have been studied in small clinical trials, and a benefit to MS was not demonstrated. Some vitamins are actually harmful if consumed in excess; these include vitamins A, D and B_6.

Salt Intake

Some of the newest information about MS and diet concerns salt. Studies in animal models of MS have reported that animals who are fed a high salt diet have worse "mouse MS" than animals fed a lower salt diet. Additionally, a recent small study of people with MS reported that people with more salt intake in their diets had a greater risk of relapse and more new and inflamed areas of nerve damage seen on their MRI scans than persons with MS who ate less salt. These findings are preliminary and need to be confirmed in larger trials, but if they are borne out, dietary salt intake may become another modifiable factor in the fight against MS.

Preventive Healthcare

Taking measures to help prevent illness is important for everyone. Preventive healthcare can enable individuals to avoid chronic illnesses such as hypertension, diabetes, obesity, lung disease, certain cancers, and heart disease. The most important preventive care tactic is to stop smoking, or to never start in the first place. The hazards of smoking have been well documented for decades, yet this highly addictive habit remains widespread. Smoking increases the risks for chronic conditions such as heart disease, lung disease, hypertension, and cancer. Smoking has been found to have numerous negative effects on bone health, including reduction in estrogen, increased free radicals, damage to bone-producing cells, and increases in cortisol, which lead to the breakdown of bone. Smoking also increases fracture risk.

For people with MS, smoking carries significant additional risks. It can worsen the disease process of MS itself and may even raise the risk of developing MS in the first place. A 2009 study by the Partners Multiple Sclerosis Center of Harvard Medical School's Brigham and Women's Hospital, the largest research effort to date looking at the relationship between smoking and MS, found that current smokers were 2.41 times more likely to have primary-progressive MS than those who had never smoked at all. The study also found that current smokers with relapsing-remitting MS advanced to secondary-progressive MS at a rate that was 2.5 times faster than nonsmokers. And a study published an April 2010 issue of *Neurology* found that among people with known risk factors for developing MS, smokers were twice as likely to develop the disease as those who had never smoked.

If you already have MS, you might wonder whether quitting smoking will actually help. The answer is yes. In the Partners study, ex-smokers progressed from relapsing-remitting to secondary-progressive MS at a rate similar to those who had never smoked at all. So by quitting smoking, you are reducing the risk that your disease will progress faster.

Obesity, which is rampant in the United States, is another important factor to consider when thinking about MS. Obesity not only increases the risks for hypertension, diabetes, and heart disease but also hampers one's ability to move about. In MS, the course of the disease often compromises mobility; individuals report such effects as weakness in their legs, poor balance, and diminished stamina. Clearly, people with MS should lose excess weight, or keep from gaining extra pounds, as that factor alone will make movement even more difficult. Newer research is beginning to uncover an association between obesity and inflammation, so other possible benefits may exist for persons with MS losing weight. In addition studies in pediatric populations indicate that childhood and adolescent obesity, particularly in girls, may also be a risk factor that increases the likelihood of developing MS.

Getting regular, thorough medical checkups, as well as routine eye and dental examinations, is also vital to preventive healthcare for everybody, including people with MS. Poor dental health may also contribute to inflammation. For women, it is additionally important to have routine gynecologic examinations. Regular breast self-exams and mammograms as well as cervical cancer screening via Pap smears are necessary for women over 40 years old. For men, testicular and prostate exams and prostate specific antigen (PSA) testing, starting at age 50, are strongly recommended.

Mental Health

Although the effects MS has on mood are covered earlier in this chapter, it is important to mention this topic again with regard to wellness-focused behaviors. Depression is a more prevalent response to MS than to any other chronic illness. As noted above, it is estimated that about 50% of people with MS will need to cope with clinical or serious depression at some time. If untreated, depression will affect social interaction, sleep, diet, cognitive function, and other aspects of living. Thus screening for depression is an important tool in preventive healthcare for people with the disease. Early identification and intervention can be very effective in managing depression successfully.

Stress Management

Many MS patients relate new symptoms, or the worsening of existing symptoms, during periods of unusual stress. For instance, Mrs. R., a 34-year-old woman with a 5-year history of MS, called her neurologist's office to report difficulty walking that began about 3 days after her mother suffered a stroke. While it is difficult to prove that the stressful event caused an increase in walking difficulty, it may have contributed to it. Stressful life events have been found to increase inflammatory substances in the blood, and this may lead to more MS activity and symptoms. Mrs. R. continued to have walking difficulties after infection was excluded as a cause for the symptoms, and she was subsequently treated with IV steroids and had improvement in her symptoms.

Stressful events and their relationship to MS have been examined in several research studies. Some results indicate that stress can increase the risk of an MS exacerbation, but others have not found a clear cause-and-effect association. Because everyone experiences stress differently—and because MS affects individuals differently—measuring its impact on symptoms of the disease is not easy. But although its effects on exacerbations are not completely clear, stress can affect mood, energy level, personal relationship health, and work performance. So it's important to make stress reduction an element of wellness-focused behaviors.

Stress-reduction activities include regular exercise, adequate rest, individual or group psychological therapy, and relaxation exercises such as meditation, tai chi, visualization, yoga, and deep breathing.

Coping with stress using such unhealthy behaviors as cigarette smoking, excessive alcohol consumption, and the use of illegal substances is generally not effective—and has obvious hazards. Patients should discuss their stress and any stress management activities, such as exercise programs, with their primary care physician and neurologist before getting started.

Personal Relationship Health

Relationships with family members and friends can surely suffer in the wake of an MS diagnosis. It is important for those with MS to realize that the diagnosis has an emotional effect on the people around them. It is difficult to "see" some of the symptoms the person with MS experiences; they may not at first grasp the impact of such symptoms.

For example, it is hard for family members to understand how MS-related fatigue can affect daily activities. "You don't look tired," is a common response. In addition, some see the fatigued individual as unmotivated and lazy. This lack of understanding can carry over to symptoms of chronic pain. Thus family members and friends need to be educated about MS and its symptoms. Through education, they likely will develop a better sense of what is being experienced and how they can help.

Over time, depending on the course of the disease, interpersonal roles in the family may be modified or changed completely. Employment can be affected, and that clearly can produce a shift in the family dynamic. Who performs certain household duties may need to change as well. These changes can produce significant conflict between family members. Discussing family issues can be difficult, but the alternative will likely lead to worsening conflict. Open communication between family members, often with the addition of family therapy, can be useful in addressing all such changes and their impact on each member of the family.

Spiritual Health

Spirituality refers to one's sensitivity or attachment to religious values and beliefs and to how one views the world because of them.

Many people participate in organized religion, some find peace and meaning through meditation, and others find their spirituality enhanced by community service and volunteering. Participating in the activities that reflect one's beliefs are ways to enhance spiritual health and are part of pursuing wellness.

Summary

Wellness encompasses all of an individual's activities and beliefs. Being diagnosed with any illness, especially a chronic disorder such as MS, can throw wellness out of balance. However, it is possible to seek and attain overall wellness through various strategies such as those discussed in this chapter. In working toward this state of being, it is important to bear in mind that wellness differs for everyone and so it is not useful for a person with MS to compare him- or herself in that regard with anyone else. Rather, it is best to concentrate on how to find one's own healthy balance among mind, body, and spirit.

Chapter 7

Reproductive Issues in Multiple Sclerosis

In this chapter, you'll learn:

- **What the effects of pregnancy are on multiple sclerosis and how multiple sclerosis affects pregnancy**
- **How multiple sclerosis treatments may affect contraception and fertility**

The majority of persons who develop MS are young adults in their 20s and 30s; over two-thirds of them are women. These are the people who are most likely to be thinking about starting or enlarging their families, and even if they are not planning on having children, they are generally sexually active. Thus questions about pregnancy, contraception, and fertility are very important. In the "bad old days," 40 or 50 years ago, women with MS were emphatically told not to have children, because there was a concern that pregnancy would worsen the disease or increase disability. Fortunately, it is now known that women with MS do very well during pregnancy; in fact sex hormones are even being explored as possible therapeutic agents to treat MS. In this chapter we will discuss the interactions between pregnancy and MS and also issues relating to contraception, fertility, and the menstrual cycle.

MS and Pregnancy

Many studies have documented that people with MS do not have increased rates of children with birth defects, nor do they have trouble getting pregnant or have other fertility problems as a result of their disease. Generally, pregnancy, labor, and delivery proceed for a woman with MS in much the same fashion as a woman in a comparable state of obstetric and general health who does not have MS. Epidural and general anesthesia are considered safe, as are cesarean sections if necessary. Generally, during pregnancy, women with MS feel well, as the immune system shifts during pregnancy to allow for the presence of the fetus. The immune system shift reduces the inflammatory activity seen in MS. Some of the symptoms of MS may be bothersome during pregnancy such a urinary frequency, difficulty in walking and fatigue, as these problems are common to any woman who is pregnant. Some women report an improvement, however, of MS symptoms during pregnancy. Most of the medications used to treat MS symptoms such as bladder problems or muscle spasticity are avoided during pregnancy because they are known to be or are possibly unsafe for the developing fetus, thus symptoms must be managed with strategies other than drugs.

Disease-Modifying Therapies

What happens to MS during pregnancy? Remember that MS represents an overactive immune system that is attacking the central nervous system. The disease-modifying agents reduce this immune response. Pregnancy acts as a natural disease-modifying entity. A baby has one set of genes and proteins from its mother and one from its father; so normally the mother's immune system would recognize the father's proteins in the developing fetus as "foreign" and attack them. But Mother Nature has cleverly engineered things so that during pregnancy the mother's immune system is modulated so it does not recognize the fetus as foreign, and the fetus is allowed to grow and develop inside the mother's body. This immune modulation turns out to be a very good thing for women with MS who become pregnant. Research has shown that during pregnancy, the relapse rate drops by two-thirds compared with what it was previous to the pregnancy. There is a brief period of several months immediately after the baby is born when the relapse rate is higher than before pregnancy, but studies have also shown that while women who become pregnant may be more likely to have a postpartum relapse, they do not have increased long-term disability compared with women with MS who do not become pregnant.

So disease-modifying therapies are not used during pregnancy. Additionally, almost all of them have been shown to cause harm to the fetus in animals or humans, so neurologists generally recommend stopping disease-modifying medications at least a month or two before a planned contraception (longer for certain drugs). If a woman does become pregnant while on a disease-modifying agent, the medication is stopped immediately.

> Jennifer and her husband go to see her neurologist. The couple has been married for about a year and is eager to start a family. Jennifer was diagnosed with MS 5 years ago and has been on beta interferon since then. She wants to have a baby but is anxious about what a pregnancy will do to her neurologic condition. The neurologist tells Jennifer and her spouse that women with MS generally have decreased relapses during pregnancy, but there is a small uptick in chances of having a relapse in the first 3 to 6 months after the baby is born. However, he reassures them that the increased risk of postpartum relapse does not appear to increase long-term disability. Additionally, Jennifer is counseled that she should stop her beta interferon for at least one menstrual period prior to attempting to conceive.

When to resume a disease-modifying medication after pregnancy is a complicated decision. Studies have shown that the women who are most likely to get a postpartum relapse are the ones who had more relapses prior to becoming pregnant, so a neurologist might advise a woman who had very active MS before she became pregnant to resume her disease-modifying therapy as soon as possible, perhaps as soon as a few weeks after the baby is born. The other factor that may determine when a woman resumes disease-modifying therapy is how long she wants to breastfeed, because these medications are not recommended in nursing mothers. These decisions should be made with input from the patient and her family, the neurologist, and the pediatrician as needed. Breastfeeding itself does not appear to increase the risk of a relapse, and a few small studies suggest that exclusive breastfeeding may even be somewhat protective against a postpartum relapse. Further research is needed in this area.

> It is now a year since Jennifer first spoke with her neurologist about pregnancy. She delivered a beautiful healthy daughter a month ago, and comes in to see the neurologist today because she has been experiencing some gait difficulty and imbalance over the past few days. The neurologist examines Jennifer and finds some new weakness in her legs. The neurologist decides to treat this relapse with a short course of intravenous steroids and some physical therapy, both of which are expected to improve Jennifer's ability to walk. Jennifer has been breastfeeding and will "pump and dump" while she is on the steroids so as not to expose the baby to them. However, both the neurologist and Jennifer are concerned about her having another relapse, and so they agree that this may be a good time for Jennifer to stop breastfeeding and resume her previous disease-modifying therapy.

As stated above, pregnancy "dials down" the immune system. There are many substances produced during pregnancy that are responsible for this, among the most powerful is a certain type of estrogen (female sex hormone) called estriol. This hormone is only produced when a woman is pregnant. Estriol has been shown to prevent or arrest disease in an animal model of MS, and in a small pilot study of 10 women with MS, reduced the inflammation that was seen on their MRIs by 80%. Estriol also appeared to protect nerves from further damage. Results of the phase 2 trial of estriol plus glatiramer acetate (GA) were reported at the annual meeting of the American Academy of Neurology in 2014. This was a multicenter trial study of 164 women with RRMS. Eighty-three were in the estriol/GA group with 60 completing 2 years. At 12 months, there were fewer relapses in the estriol/GA group compared to the GA alone group. Improvements were also seen in the cognitive test scores of those in the estriol/GA group. Testosterone, the main male sex hormone, has also been shown to have neuroprotective effects in animal studies and a small human study, and further investigation with this hormone is ongoing as well.

Currently there are no prenatal tests that can indicate whether a child whose parent or sibling has MS will develop the disease. Remember that the risk of developing MS in a first-degree relative of someone with MS is about 4%.

Other Reproductive Issues

Persons with MS may use any form of contraception, but some of the medicines used for symptom management, particularly some of the anticonvulsing drugs used to treat pain, and stimulants such as modafinil may interfere with hormonal contraception (the "pill"), so it is a good idea to discuss this with your doctor.

Some women with MS may experience an increase in some of their neurologic symptoms right before their menstrual periods, which resolve as soon as the period starts. It is not known what produces this increase in symptoms; sometimes hormones are used to regulate the periods to prevent this increased symptom activity.

The effects of menopause on MS have not been well studied at all. At this time there are no data to indicate that taking hormone replacement to relieve menopausal symptoms is beneficial or harmful to those with MS.

Summary

People with MS do not have an increased incidence of birth defects or infertility. Pregnancy, labor, and delivery are usually conducted in the same way as for a woman who does not have MS. Pregnancy itself has a beneficial effect on relapses, and the slightly higher relapse rate seen in the first few months after the baby is born has not been shown to increased long-term disability. Disease-modifying agents are not recommended for use during pregnancy or breastfeeding and should be stopped before a planned pregnancy.

Chapter 8

The Future of Multiple
Sclerosis Management

In this chapter, you'll learn:

- **How research trials are conducted**
- **What the different types of stem cells are and how they may be used to repair damaged nerves**
- **What other new research initiatives are on the horizon**

In the preceding chapters we've defined what multiple sclerosis (MS) is and how one goes about managing the myriad of symptoms and potential challenges presented by disease. Since the 1990s we have seen rapid advances in our understanding of and ability to manage MS. Obviously, though, there is still much room for improvement. In this chapter, we'll take a look at where research is headed.

How Is Research Conducted?

Most treatments for human diseases get their start in a laboratory, tested in cells and/or animals. For example, a condition that bears similarity to MS (experimental allergic encephalomyelitis, or EAE) can be induced in mice or rats, and most MS drugs are first tested in this animal model. Once a drug or compound has been shown to be safe and effective in this setting, trials in humans can commence, starting with a "phase 1" trial. Phase 1 trials are conducted in a small number of people, for example, 10 to 15, and may consist of healthy volunteers or people who have the disease or condition for which the drug is being studied. Phase 1 trials are done to establish the safety and the appropriate dose range and the drug side effects. If the drug appears to be safe in humans in this small study, then phase 2 trials are planned. A phase 2 trial is generally conducted to further evaluate safety and to begin to look at efficacy in a random-ized, blinded, controlled fashion with up to a few hundred subjects. What does this entail?

Randomization assigns each subject to a treatment intervention by a process similar to flipping a coin. This ensures that each treat-ment group has the same number and type of subjects, for example, equal numbers of men and women, equal numbers of people in each group who may be using a cane to walk, or other criteria that are being studied.

Blinding means that ideally neither the investigator nor the sub-jects know which type of treatment individual subjects are receiving ("double blind"). This is to avoid any bias that might influence the results.

Having a control group for a trial is very important. This means that the group of subjects receiving the drug or treatment under investigation is matched with a similar group of subjects who get either a known standard drug or a placebo (inactive substance). Sometimes a trial will have an investigational arm, a standard treatment arm, and a placebo arm, or different doses of the inves-tigational treatment versus standard drug or placebo. These con-trols are particularly important when testing treatments for MS, because very often people with MS improve spontaneously, and one has to demonstrate that improvement due to an investiga-tional treatment would not have happened by chance, but is really due to the treatment. This is one reason why anecdotal reports of supposed treatments or "cures" for MS have to be viewed very critically if they are just based on personal testimony and not con-trolled trials.

If the phase 2 trials are successful, then phase 3 trials, which involve many hundreds of subjects at multiple sites, are done. For trials in MS, it generally takes at least 2 years to see an effect of a treatment. The investigation process from the laboratory through phase 3 clinical trials takes several years, but is very important to learn as much as possible (both safety and efficacy) about the treatment before it is approved for general use.

Scientists are working diligently on unraveling the mysteries of the genetics, immunology, and epidemiology of MS. Through this research, more effective and more convenient treatment options that involve fewer side effects will be discovered. Stopping MS progression and reversing the damage it causes remain the ultimate goals.

Both genetics and the environment appear to play a role in the development of MS. Genetics research has shown that numerous genes, perhaps 200 or more, may contribute to the risk of MS. Other genes also have been identified that may offer protection from the development of MS. Many of these genes appear to help regulate immune responses in the human body. A better understanding of these genetic factors may aid in the earlier diagnosis of MS and may also help guide treatment choices. For example, genetic biomarkers may enable us to predict which therapy will be best suited to a given individual.

But genetics alone does not tell the whole story. In identical twins, if one twin has MS, the likelihood of the other having MS is about 30%. If genes alone were to blame, the risk of MS in that other twin would be 100%—so clearly, other factors are involved.

The environment appears to also play a role in MS. Research has shown that viruses such as the Epstein-Barr virus (EBV) are associated with the risk of developing MS. Developing a viral infection in childhood versus adulthood seems to be important and more likely associated with the later development of MS. Vitamin D levels and childhood sunlight exposure also appear to contribute to the risk of MS. In addition, childhood and adolescent obesity may be a risk factor for MS. Based on data from clinical trials, cigarette smoking is believed to be another risk factor for the development of MS. Researchers are looking at how these factors may be manipulated to lower the risk of MS and potentially alter the course of MS.

These complicated genetic and environmental factors come together to result in an altered immune response for the person with MS. This faulty immune response drives the inflammatory process which causes demyelination and damage to axons (nerve fibers) in the brain and spinal cord.

The current disease-modifying agents for MS are very effective anti-inflammatory treatments, and their use results in fewer relapses, fewer new lesions detected by MRI, and slowed progression of disability. However, it is important to know that these agents are *treatments* and not a cure for MS. While they are highly effective for many persons with MS, for some, they are not as effective. And most of these agents require self-injection.

Numerous drugs that may be more effective and easier to administer are in clinical trials. Several orally administered therapies are now available, and others are being tested. Other types of injectable drugs are in development and they may be equally or more effective than currently available options. As new therapies become available, people with MS and their healthcare providers will need to take a hard look at not only the convenience and efficacy but also the safety of any new options.

Stem cells may play a role in stopping the progression of MS and reversing the damage. **Stem cells** are defined as cells that can replicate themselves or differentiate into many cell types. These properties make them interesting to researchers looking to repair or replace damaged cells or tissue in the human body. Stem cells can be divided into embryonic stem cells and adult stem cells. The former have the potential to develop into any of the body's cell types, while adult stem cells may be limited to producing only certain types of cells. While many of us think of stem cells as having the ability to regenerate damaged myelin and nerve fibers, stem cell research has other possibilities.

Sites around the world are researching the use of hematopoietic stem cell transplantation (HSCT) for MS. The question is, If a person with MS has an immune system that has "learned" to attack myelin as a result of genetic and environmental influences, might it be possible to just "reboot" the immune system?

Adult stem cells, called hematopoietic stem cells, are obtained from the patient's bone marrow or blood and are saved. The person is then treated with high doses of immunosuppressive drugs (chemotherapy) so that their immune system is "ablated" or shut down. The saved stem cells are then administered to the patient. These cells have not "learned" to have MS. Early trials have shown some success in shutting down inflammation and relapses in people with aggressive forms of MS. This procedure has not been shown to reverse established disability, however. Furthermore, HSCT is not without risks, and deaths have occurred from the procedure. It is also important to note that hematopoietic stem cells can also be obtained from umbilical cord blood.

Mesenchymal stem cells are adult stem cells that typically differentiate (develop into) into bone, fat, muscle, or tendons. Animal research has shown that these cells may also have the potential to develop into neural tissue and to reduce inflammation in the immune system. The appeal of these mesenchymal stem cells is that they are readily available. Cells can be obtained from bone marrow and adult fat, (which, unfortunately, many of us have plenty of). These cells may hold promise for future MS treatment. Further trials are currently in progress.

When many people think of stem cells, they think of embryonic stem cells. Embryonic stem cells are typically obtained from unused embryos that are the result of in vitro fertilization (IVF). This practice has led to ethical concerns and debates about this source of embryonic stem cells. Another potential source of stem cells is through a process called nuclear transfer. This procedure creates embryonic stem cells by injecting the nucleus with all the genetic material from an adult cell, like a skin cell, into an unfertilized human egg that has had its nucleus removed. This process has been successful in creating animal embryonic stem cells, but not human ones yet.

Embryonic stem cells do hold the promise of repairing damage in the central nervous system such as is seen with MS because they can (theoretically) be manipulated into becoming any type of cell that is desired. Many challenges remain, however. Embryonic stem cells have been associated with the development of undesired tissues in both animal and human trials.

Researchers are looking at transplanting embryonic stem cells directly into injured tissue—something that has been done with spinal cord trauma. These oligodendrocyte (myelin-forming cells) precursor cells (OPCs) then mature into myelin-producing cells, with the hope that they will repair damaged myelin and produce more myelin, improving function. But unlike with spinal cord trauma, people with MS have multiple sites of damage, so this approach could be more challenging for this condition. Some research is suggesting that embryonic stem cells could be injected into the cerebrospinal fluid or bloodstream and that the cells will "home in" on the damaged tissue where they are needed. This approach would be more applicable to the person with MS.

Other potential sources for repair of myelin in the central nervous system are Schwann cells (which produce myelin in peripheral nerves) and olfactory nerve–ensheathing cells. While these are not stem cells, both produce myelin and are being looked at for their repair potential. Thus far, success has been limited by poor survival of the cells after transplantation and the need to transplant the cells directly into damaged tissue.

A word of caution is warranted when discussing stem cell therapies for MS. Legitimate research is ongoing, including clinical trials for some of the different types of stem cells described above. Numerous for-profit clinics have popped up worldwide offering cures for a wide range of conditions, including MS. While progressive forms of MS can leave a person feeling desperate for a definitive treatment, these clinics are definitely a lesson in "buyer beware." Most are located in countries that do not have the same strict standards for regulation and patient safety that are present in the United States and have no data from properly controlled trials that prove that their therapies are effective. Use caution when investigating clinics which promise a "cure" not only for MS but also for a variety of conditions.

In addition to cells that may play a role in neural repair, numerous substances exist that either promote or inhibit myelin growth in the human nervous system. Researchers are examining the potential for modifying these substances to promote repair. Ultimately, the answer may come from a combination of both cell transplants and the use of compounds to enhance remyelination and cell survival.

Finally, researchers are also focusing on the role of rehabilitation in helping people with MS improve function and adapt to the challenges of MS. Active participation in exercise may help promote the rerouting of electrical pathways in the central nervous system of the person with MS. Many studies in animals have indicated that exercise can help to stimulate the formation of new nerve connections, increase some nerve growth factors, and decrease the production of some inflammatory substances. Trials in people with MS have shown that exercise may improve some symptoms, such as fatigue, depression, and spasticity, and in some cases may lead to improved muscle strength and mobility. In addition, ongoing trials are investigating whether exercise can improve the ability to think and remember in persons with cognitive difficulties due to MS. Technologic advances are also being made in assistive devices such as electronic stimulators to overcome muscle weakness and robotic devices that fit over weakened legs and help them to walk.

Summary

It is more than possible to live well with MS. To achieve this goal, it's important to strike a balance, integrating knowledge of current resources with a comprehensive and multidisciplinary healthcare team and a watchful eye on the horizon as research advances.

Chapter 9

Planning for Your Future

Managing Your Personal Affairs

We all know in theory that we should plan for unexpected family emergencies, such as a stroke or a car accident. When diagnosed with MS, we know that we should make plans to allow us to live as independently as possible for as long as possible. Day-to-day matters often allow us to push this kind of planning to the bottom of our "to do" list, however. Planning for emergencies by necessity involves difficult family discussions that we might prefer to avoid. Addressing difficult family decisions before an emergency arises—and before your MS progresses to where you no longer are able to participate in decision-making makes it much easier for your loved ones to assist you through the emergency because you will have stated how you want your affairs handled. To illustrate, consider the following example:

> John visited his aging mother, Bertha, and they discussed the importance of an advance directive and a power of attorney. Bertha insisted that she did not want the family to take any unusual life-prolonging measures if something were to happen so that she could not make decisions for herself. She asked that John handle her finances if she were to become unable to do so. After this conversation, John made an appointment with his mother's attorney, and after several
>
> *(Continued)*

(Continued)

more discussions among the three of them, Bertha decided to sign an advance directive and a durable power of attorney. A month later, Bertha had a severe stroke that did in fact leave her unable to communicate.

If John had not started this discussion with his mother about an advance directive and power of attorney, Bertha's other children might never have learned about her end-of-life wishes. Had John and Bertha not taken the time to have an advance directive and power of attorney discussed, drafted, and signed, John would not have been able to handle even routine financial matters for his mother after her stroke.

This chapter explains the importance of planning for the future *and* provides useful information to assist you and your family with these details. You will learn ways to ensure that your affairs are managed as you want them to be managed—even if you are no longer able to communicate or make decisions yourself.

You will learn about the following:

- Informal arrangements with friends or family
- Formal arrangements with or without court involvement
  - To manage your financial affairs such as powers of attorney, trusts, and conservatorships
  - To manage your healthcare through healthcare directives, living wills, POLSTs (Physician Orders for Life Sustaining Treatments), DNR/DNI/DNHs (Do Not Resuscitate/Do Not Intubate/Do Not Hospitalize), or guardianships
  - To ensure that your postdeath wishes are followed regarding your property and the disposition of your body

Your Emergency Notebook

A first step in planning for emergencies is assembling and maintaining key health, financial, and other information in one place so that family members and caregivers may access the information if you are suddenly unable to communicate with them. Many organizations have developed planning guides that are free for members. But you can also create your own "emergency notebook" with a three-ring binder and a set of divider tabs—or on your computer. If you have all of your information on your computer or other electronic device, make sure that the person who will be acting as your agent knows all of your passwords and where the information is stored. For both types of notebooks, it's a good idea to go over the information with your agent while you have capacity. Organize your emergency notebook as follows, with tabs or separate folders for separating documents and information into the following sections:

1. Emergency contact information
   - Spouse, partner, or significant other
   - Children
   - Siblings
   - Parents
2. Financial and legal contact information
   - Estate attorney
   - Accountant
   - Investment advisor
3. Medical information
   - Medication (recent, past, and present)
   - Contact information for both primary care and specialist physicians
   - Immunization records
   - Significant medical, dental, and eye care details (including the physicians' names and locations of medical records)
   - Allergies
   - Significant family medical history

4. Financial information
   - Bank accounts
   - Insurance policies
   - Retirement plans
   - Stocks and bonds
   - Recurring bills (for example: utilities, insurance, mortgage payments)
   - Real and personal property
   - Loans (receivable and payable)
   - Financial powers of attorney
   - Taxes (location of past tax returns and information for current tax year)
   - Safe deposit box
5. End-of-life information
   - Will and any accompanying statement concerning final arrangements for personal property
   - Advance directive
   - Organ donor information
   - Funeral and burial guidance
6. Location of key items
   - Important documents (for example: passports, military records, deeds, marriage license, Social Security numbers, titles to vehicles)
   - Photos
   - Jewelry
7. Passwords and electronic media (Passwords are vital, and given that they frequently change, don't forget to update your emergency notebook, even if by hand.)
   - Home and office computers
   - Software programs
   - Financial and medical websites
   - Facebook and similar pages (consider, for instance, how you want these handled after your death)

Of course, an emergency notebook is not helpful if family members cannot find or access it. It must be stored in a safe place—but you must let trusted individuals know where the notebook and electronic information are located.

Informal and Formal Arrangements

A second step in planning is to make arrangements for events that may be anticipated or unanticipated. Depending on the circumstance, the arrangements made will be either informal or formal.

Informal Care Arrangements

Informal arrangements are temporary and can usually be made with family, friends, and neighbors. For example, if you have surgery scheduled or you are experiencing a lot of fatigue and know that you will be unable to perform normal household chores either while you are recuperating or for the indefinite future, you may want to line up family members or friends to assist with your medication, grocery shopping, cooking, transportation to medical appointments, or housekeeping. You may also want them to help with financial matters, such as writing out checks, filling out tax returns, and balancing the checkbook. Such informal arrangements are very common and, in fact, make up the majority of assistance to people who are temporarily or permanently living with disabilities.

Entrusting private financial or medical information to family members or friends, however, may have unintended negative consequences. It may result in uncomfortable situations that may even have financially or medically harmful consequences. In such cases, formal arrangements are preferable. Formal arrangements may include legal safeguards regarding supervision and record-keeping or review by an outside party to minimize the risk of exploitation by an informal caregiver. Similarly, formal arrangements may also be made to protect the caregiver, who might later be questioned regarding legitimate reimbursement for services.

Even when informal arrangements work well, the day may come when more formal arrangements are needed.

Formal Financial Management Services

When planning for the future, it is important to know what financial management services are available for your individual needs. These services are listed next, starting from the least to the most formal.

Automatic Banking and Direct Deposit

Modern banking technology, such as automatic bill payment and direct deposit, can help you with your finances. At a minimum, Social Security payments and pension income should be set up so they are directly deposited. Utilities and insurance payments should also be set up to be withdrawn automatically from your account. Doing so can prevent you from unintentionally discontinuing your health insurance or from having your electricity shut off. It is wise to have one "working" bank account, such as a checking account, into which income is deposited and from which monthly bills are paid.

To arrange for Social Security checks to be deposited directly to a bank account, you may call Social Security at 1–800–772–1213 and ask for a direct deposit form or sign up on the Social Security Direct Deposit page online at http://www.ssa.gov/deposit/. A bank can also provide you with this form. Beginning March 1, 2013, all Social Security recipients are, with limited exceptions, required to have checks directly deposited.

Multiple-Name Bank Accounts

Adding a name to a bank account is an easy and effective way to allow a trusted relative or friend to provide informal help. By having access to the account, that person can help sign checks, pay bills, or transfer money between your accounts. That person can also have access to bank records to monitor electronic deposits, ensure that all bills are paid on time, and review monthly statements to ensure that nothing is amiss in all your accounts.

Several types of multiple-name bank accounts are available, each with different rules. Any type of account—for example, savings, checking, and certificates of deposit—may be held in more than one name. Such accounts are easy to set up just by visiting the bank. However, great care must be taken to select the appropriate type of account (as explained next) for your situation and to assure that you have selected a trustworthy person to help you.

The following types of multiple-name accounts are commonly available:

Joint Account
In a joint account, any person whose name is on the account is considered a co-owner. Each named person can make deposits and withdrawals without the other person's knowledge or consent. There are a few facts about joint accounts to keep in mind:

- The other person could withdraw all of your money without consequence or legal recourse.
- The other person's creditors could tie up the funds in the account (with a lien or attachment) until proof of your ownership of the funds is provided.
- A person's name cannot be taken off the account without that person's written approval.
- In a joint account, when one owner dies, the survivor automatically owns the account without going through

probate court. This can be a benefit because the funds are immediately available to pay urgent expenses, such as funeral costs. It can also have negative consequences if the joint account holder is not your intended beneficiary.

Authorized Signer Account

An authorized signer account, or a convenience account, allows another individual to make deposits and withdrawals to your account and sign your checks. The other signer's creditors cannot tie up your account. As with joint accounts, however, there is still the risk that the other authorized signer could withdraw all your money from your account. Unlike a joint account, the account does not belong to the other authorized signer upon your death; rather, funds in this account belong to your estate—or to a named beneficiary (see below). The authority of the other signer ends with your death, so the other authorized signer will not be able to use the funds after your death.

Payable on Death Accounts and Beneficiary Designations

All checking, savings, investment, and retirement accounts allow you to designate to whom your account will be distributed at your death. Sometimes these accounts are called payable on death (POD) or transfer on death (TOD) accounts. Both the beneficiary designation and the POD/TOD account allow for planning after your death, but these designations do not affect ownership during your life. The named beneficiary cannot make withdrawals or sign checks, so it is a useful way to bypass probate to give money to loved ones after your death.

Naming a Representative Payee

A representative payee is an individual or organization appointed by the US Social Security Administration, the US Office of Personnel Management, the US Department of Veterans Affairs, or the US

Railroad Retirement Board who may be charged with receiving your income, using that income to pay your current expenses, saving for your future needs, and maintaining proper records. The Social Security Administration has a Representative Payee Program with rules and regulations to protect the beneficiary of the income. Learn more about the Representative Payee Program at http://www .socialsecurity.gov/payee. To have the authority to manage your Social Security or Supplemental Security Income benefit, a person or organization must be appointed by the Social Security Administration. A power of attorney or note from you is not good enough. Having a representative appointed provides oversight that may give you assurance that your bills and finances will be properly handled. Many professional fiduciaries and organizations serve as representative payees.

Family Caregiving Contracts
Individuals are often uncomfortable with the idea of paying family members or friends for caregiving arrangements. But changes in the Medicaid asset transfer rules since the early 2000s, as well as the reality that caregivers must sometimes give up their day jobs in order to provide the necessary level of care, have made personal care contracts an attractive option, to make sure both that the level of care is met and that children (or other relatives or friends) do not have to sacrifice their own financial well-being while providing care to their parents or loved ones.

Personal care contracts must, as a general rule, be in writing and state the kind and extent of services that are necessary, within reasonable terms. Because personal services contracts involve payment for services, income paid to a family caregiver through such a contract is subject to payroll and income taxes, and caregivers should consult an accountant to ensure that the income is reported properly. Tax credits are not available for parent caregiving unless the parent is the child's legal dependent.

Durable Power of Attorney

A power of attorney is an extremely important planning tool. It allows you to appoint someone to manage all or some of your financial affairs if you are unable to manage them yourself. If no power of attorney exists and it is necessary to liquidate or transfer assets or enter into real estate transactions (including those of a spouse), it may be necessary to go to court to establish a conservatorship before these matters can be acted on. Establishing a conservatorship can be costly and time-consuming. Thus, everyone should have a power of attorney.

Power of Attorney Defined

A **power of attorney** is a written document in which you (as the "principal") appoint another person (the "attorney-in-fact") to handle your property or finances. The power of attorney can be effective for all purposes or for a limited purpose (for example, appointing another person to sign a deed for the sale of your home when you are unavailable). A power of attorney becomes ineffective if the principal becomes incapacitated or dies.

Durable Power of Attorney Defined

A "durable" power of attorney continues to be valid even after the principal becomes incapacitated. A durable power of attorney document must specifically state that it is "durable" and must contain specific language, such as "This power of attorney shall continue to be effective if I become incapacitated or incompetent." Generally, if the purpose of a power of attorney is to make sure that someone can manage your finances when you cannot, the power of attorney should be durable.

Care Must Be Taken in Choosing an Attorney-in-Fact

Powers of attorney are not supervised by courts, so they can be abused if the wrong person is appointed attorney-in-fact. While the attorney-in-fact is required by law to act in the best interest of the principal, it is difficult to get your money back if the person you have appointed handles your affairs unwisely. Therefore, you must choose someone you trust implicitly—a person who will *always* act in your best interests.

Creating a Power of Attorney

While forms are available free on the Internet, it is best to consult an experienced attorney to create a power of attorney. Too many times, individuals sign documents they have printed off the Internet only to discover later that the documents are invalid or do not serve their purposes. This can be a very costly error, because it may be necessary to have a court appoint a conservator to do what could have been accomplished easily with a validly executed power of attorney.

Safeguards to Protect You

You may trust a friend or family member to be your attorney-in-fact and feel confident that no safeguards are necessary. However, another option is to hire a professional fiduciary, such as a bank trust department, to ensure that your finances are handled the way you want. Either way, consider including the following safeguards in a power of attorney:

- Require that the attorney-in-fact provide an annual or monthly accounting to you, your lawyer, an independent accountant, or a trusted family member to review.

- Name two attorneys-in-fact on the document and specify that they must act jointly (for example, both attorneys-infact must agree and both must sign checks).
- Require your appointed attorney-in-fact to obtain a surety bond to cover the value of your property if the attorney-in-fact mishandles your funds.
- Appoint a successor in case the attorney-in-fact dies, becomes incompetent, or simply chooses not to act on your behalf.

Cancelling or Ending a Power of Attorney

A power of attorney can be canceled or revoked at any time. Each state has specific requirements for revoking a power of attorney. Your revocation should be sent to the attorney-in-fact and to any person or institution with whom the attorney-in-fact has done business on your behalf.

Remember, a power of attorney becomes invalid if the principal becomes incompetent or dies. A *durable* power of attorney continues if the principal becomes incompetent and can be revoked only by a guardian or conservator, if one has been appointed. A durable power of attorney terminates when the principal dies.

Trusts

A trust is a legal arrangement in which a person or a financial institution owns and manages assets for your benefit. The parties to a trust are the person setting up the trust (the "grantor"), the person or organization administering the trust (the "trustee"), and the person for whom the trust is established (the "beneficiary"). Often the grantor and the beneficiary are the same person.

An agreement, called a trust instrument, between the grantor and the trustee explains the trustee's authority. A trust can be created by the terms of the grantor's will (a **testamentary trust**) or during the grantor's lifetime (a **living trust**, also called an inter vivos trust). A living trust is the type of trust used to manage assets during a time of incapacity. Some trusts are court supervised, and some are not.

Trusts are not for everyone. A living trust is generally not appropriate for modest estates because the costs and disadvantages, including the time and logistics involved in administering them, outweigh the benefits. As with any planning tool, it is important to review each option for managing estates to determine the strategies that best fit your situation. In other words, one size does not fit all.

Basic Living Trust Defined

You may create a living trust during your lifetime by transferring ownership and control of your assets to the trust.

A trust can be revocable or irrevocable:

- As long as you are competent, you may change, revoke, or terminate a **revocable trust** at any time during your lifetime. A revocable trust is normally used for property management purposes. After you die, the revocable trust becomes irrevocable.
- A revocable living trust is often used as a planning tool because it allows a trustee to manage your property for your benefit during life and can also provide for distribution or ongoing management after your incapacity or death. Most commonly, in a living trust you would be both your own trustee and beneficiary. As such, your Social Security number would be used when establishing trust accounts or doing trust business. You would manage your property as if the property were in your name. A trust agreement would also include your directions should you become incompetent or die. If you have a medical condition that could result in your being unable to manage your affairs, a revocable living trust may be the right choice.

- An **irrevocable trust** cannot be changed or terminated after it has been established. It is a separate taxable entity, requiring its own tax identification number. Tax considerations may be a factor in deciding whether to make a trust revocable or irrevocable, particularly when a substantial amount of property is involved.

Care Must Be Taken in Choosing a Trustee

A trustee has as much, if not more, responsibility as an attorney-in-fact in a power of attorney. Great care must be taken in choosing your trustee. In most revocable living trusts, you would serve as trustee as long as you are able to do so. Should you become incapacitated, the "successor trustee" would take over and be responsible for management of all trust assets during your life and for distribution of those assets to the beneficiaries upon your death. Being a trustee is a huge responsibility and should not be taken lightly. While a family member or other individual could be named trustee if you are sure that person is trustworthy and capable of acting in this capacity, a fair amount of expertise is needed to handle the paperwork, tax returns, and property management tasks that may be involved. In most cities, professional trustees are available for hire, and many banking institutions have trust departments. Going over options with an attorney before naming a trustee is always wise.

Creating a Living Trust

A revocable living trust is established with the execution of a trust agreement. In this document, you would name the beneficiary (usually yourself during life), state how the property should be managed if you become disabled, and direct how the property should be distributed at your death. A living trust is much like a will in this way, and so many states require specific formalities in signing a trust to ensure that you are not being coerced or unduly influenced by someone in executing the trust. Trusts should be drawn up by an attorney familiar with drafting them.

Important Tip

Be on guard against anyone who uses high-pressure tactics to sell a living trust package. Do not deal with anyone who demands a signature right away or requires money before you have time to do additional research. Some companies only want to sell their prepackaged plans and do not assist clients in putting assets into the trust. These trusts can cause problems that are expensive to fix.

To receive the advantages of the revocable trust, all assets must be placed in the trust or the trust must be named beneficiary.

A Revocable Trust Cannot Be Used to Avoid Paying Nursing Home Costs

A revocable trust is considered an available resource under Medicaid laws and is not a way to avoid spending savings on nursing home care. The federal and state Medicaid laws are very complicated and subject to change at any time. Do not try to use a trust without getting competent legal advice.

Trusts for Protecting Assets While Dependent on Medicaid

People living with chronic conditions may ultimately require assistance with activities of daily living (ADLs), such as bathing, transferring, ambulation, eating, toileting, and basic hygiene and grooming. This type of assistance is known as custodial care. Individuals may receive this care at home, or they may need to move to an assisted living facility or a nursing home. No matter where these services are received, they are very expensive. Medicare does not cover the cost of custodial care. Long-term care insurance policies may cover these types of costs. It is difficult to obtain long-term care insurance after you are diagnosed with a significant medical condition. When long-term care insurance is not available, private funds must be used to pay for the cost of care. Once private funds are depleted, many individuals turn to Medicaid to pay for these services.

Medicaid eligibility rules are complex and vary depending on (among other things) the state in which you reside, whether you are married or single, the types of services you need, and your age. As a very general rule, however, you may keep a car and your home (as long as you are living in it) and about $3,000. Be aware that this amount varies from state to state. The point is, you can have only limited assets outside of your home and car. There are three types of trusts available that, if properly established and administered, allow a person with a disability to retain more than $3,000 and still be eligible for Medicaid to pay for the cost of care. These three trusts are a first-party special needs trust; a third-party special needs trust, and a pooled trust. The funds in any of these three trusts may be used to purchase goods and/ or services that "supplement and do not supplant" government benefits. In other words, funds in the trust may be used for goods and/or services that benefit the individual and do not replace the government benefits the individual receives. For instance, funds may be used to pay for a companion dog, nonconventional treatments, massage, companion services, a home, rent, travel, or clothing. Funds may not be used to pay for medical services covered by Medicaid. Because you can have only $3,000 to be eligible for Medicaid to pay the cost of custodial care, having a special needs trust can make a significant difference in your life. Sometimes a special needs trust can make the difference between living at home or in a nursing home.

First-Party Special Needs Trust

A first-party special needs trust is a way for an individual to place his or her own money into a trust and remain eligible for Medicaid. It is called a "first-party" special needs trust because the individual's assets are used to fund the trust. Assets in a first-party special needs trust remain exempt if:

- The trust is established by a parent, grandparent, guardian, or court and is for the sole benefit of the individual—the beneficiary—who is under the age of 65 and who has been certified disabled by the Social Security Administration.
  - The trust is funded with the individual's assets—for instance savings or assets awarded as a result of a personal injury lawsuit.
- The trust is irrevocable and may only be changed by the trustee if the change is necessary to comply with a new law or decision governing first-party special needs trusts.
- The trust has a provision that at the death of the individual with the disability, any remaining trust assets must be distributed first to the State Medicaid Agency in an amount equal to the total amount of Medicaid paid on behalf of the individual.

Third-Party Special Needs Trust

A third-party special needs trust is a way for a third party to give money to an individual with a disability in a way that does not jeopardize the individual's eligibility for public benefits. For instance, if a parent or grandparent or best friend wants to leave money to an individual with a disability, or if friends want to throw a fund-raiser, a third-party special needs trust is used. Sometimes third-party trusts are set up while the grantor is alive; other times they are set up in wills. Assets or funds belonging to the person with the disability must never be placed in the trust. There is no payback to the State Medicaid Agency. Rather, the grantor may state who will receive any funds remaining in trust at the beneficiary's death. Laws regarding the supplemental needs trusts vary from state to state, and a lawyer should be consulted in each state.

Pooled Trust

A pooled trust is a type of special needs trust, and for all intents and purposes it is administered like a first-party special needs trust except that a pooled trust must be established and managed by a nonprofit corporation. A separate subaccount must be maintained for each beneficiary of the trust, but, for purposes of investment and management, the trust pools the accounts. Each subaccount must be established solely for the benefit of individuals who are disabled as defined by the Social Security Administration. The subaccount may be set up by the parent, grandparent, or legal guardian of the individual, the individual him- or herself, or by a court. To the extent that amounts remaining in the subaccount at the beneficiary's death are not retained by the pooled trust, the trust must pay such remaining amounts to the state in an amount equal to the total amount of Medicaid paid on behalf of the individual.

Healthcare Directives

A healthcare directive, often called an advance directive, is a written document in which you appoint someone (a healthcare agent) to make healthcare decisions in the event you are unable to make them yourself.

A healthcare directive is now recognized as a combination of two earlier documents: the living will (a document that provides specific guidance to physicians, nurses, and caregivers about medical treatment) and a durable power of attorney for healthcare (a document that authorizes another person to make healthcare decisions when you are unable to do so).

Why Create a Healthcare Directive?

You have the right to make decisions about your healthcare, including the right to refuse treatment, authorize treatment, and access information in your medical records. In a healthcare directive, you can authorize an agent—usually a trusted loved one, relative, or caregiver to make necessary healthcare decisions according to your wishes if you are unable to do so yourself.

What Must a Healthcare Directive Include?

Healthcare directives are governed by state law, and most state laws have several statutory requirements. Most important, a healthcare directive must be written by a competent person, and be dated, signed, and witnessed or notarized.

Who Can Be a Healthcare Agent?

Your healthcare agent may be any individual 18 years of age or older who is not your healthcare provider or an employee of your healthcare provider. You should choose someone who you know well and trust to make decisions according to your wishes. It is very important to discuss your wishes in detail with a prospective healthcare agent before you finalize your decision. Make sure the person clearly understands your wishes *and* appreciates the responsibilities involved. You should also name a successor (backup) healthcare agent in case the primary healthcare agent is unable to act when decisions must be made.

What Is Included in the Healthcare Directive?

In your healthcare directive, you may:

- Appoint one or more agents or alternative agents and include instructions for how decisions should be made and whether named agents must act together or may act independently
- State a preferred nursing home in the event such care is necessary
- State which medical records the healthcare agent can access
- State that the healthcare agent is the "personal representative" under the federal Health Insurance Portability and Accountability Act (HIPAA) and has the authority to access your medical records
- State whether the healthcare agent shall be guardian or conservator if a petition is filed
- State whether your eyes, tissues, or organs should be donated on your death
- Make a declaration regarding intrusive mental health treatment or a statement that the healthcare agent is authorized to give consent for such treatment
- State specific instructions if you are female and pregnant
- Give instructions regarding artificially administered nutrition or hydration
- State under what circumstances the healthcare directive will become effective
- State any other instructions regarding care, including how religious beliefs may affect healthcare delivery

- Provide instructions about being placed on a ventilator, receiving resuscitation, or other aggressive measures if there is minimal to no chance that you will recover
- State what will happen with your body at death (body identification/burial/cremation)

When Do the Healthcare Agent's Responsibilities Begin?

Generally, the healthcare agent may make decisions for you when your physician believes you are unable to make your own decisions.

What Are the Duties of the Healthcare Agent?

The healthcare agent is obligated to make informed, good-faith healthcare decisions from your point of view. The healthcare agent should follow your guidance in the healthcare directive and should seek legal help if the medical providers will not comply with his or her requests.

Can the Healthcare Directive Be Cancelled or Revoked?

You may cancel or revoke the healthcare directive in whole or in part by:

- Destroying the document
- Executing a written and dated statement explaining what part of the healthcare directive you want to revoke
- Verbally expressing the intent to revoke it in the presence of witnesses
- Executing a new healthcare directive

Where Should the Healthcare Directive Be Kept?

The healthcare directive must be readily available in an emergency. It should be kept with your personal papers in a safe place—such as your emergency notebook—(not in a safe deposit box unless someone else is also a signer on the box). You should give signed copies to family members, close friends, your healthcare agent, your backup healthcare agent, and your doctors so that they can include it in your medical records.

What Is the Uniform Anatomical Gift Act?

The Uniform Anatomical Gift Act allows you to donate your entire body, organs, tissues, or eyes for research or transplantation. If you do not make the gift, close relatives, a guardian, a conservator, or a healthcare agent may make an anatomical gift at the time of death—unless you documented while you were alive that you do not want to donate your organs. Verification of intent to make an anatomical gift may be indicated on your driver's license.

Is a DNR/DNI/DNH the Same as a Healthcare Directive?

The acronym DNR/DNI/DNH means "do not resuscitate/do not intubate/do not hospitalize." This is a request by a patient to his or her physician to limit the scope of emergency medical care. The request is signed by the patient or the patient's proxy, and it must be ordered by a physician. It will be followed by emergency medical personnel if presented to them at the time of the emergency. You should have a healthcare directive as well, because the DNR/DNI/DNH is limited only to decisions regarding the end of life and resuscitation or intubation and does not deal with all other myriad issues that may arise at the end of one's life.

What Is POLST and Is It the Same as a Healthcare Directive?

The acronym "POLST" stands for Physician Orders for Life-Sustaining Treatment. The POLST paradigm is the product of an initiative that began in Oregon in 1991 in recognition that patient wishes for life-sustaining treatments were not being honored despite the availability of advance directives. As of August 2014, the National POLST Paradigm Task Force had endorsed and was developing programs in about 43 states. The individual POLST programs develop medical orders that can be used by emergency medical technicians and other healthcare professionals during an emergency. The POLST form is more specific than an advance directive and is signed by the patient's provider, making it a medical order. The physician must meet with the patient or a surrogate to go over the form and learn treatment options available for the specific disease or serious illness the patient has. Like the DNR/DNI/DNH order, the POLST form is not meant to take the place of an advance directive or the appointment of the agent.

Where Can I Obtain Healthcare Directive Forms?

An attorney who specializes in eldercare law or has experience with healthcare directives can prepare a directive that is tailored to your needs.

In addition, suitable forms may be downloaded from reputable websites, such as the following:

- Aging with Dignity: *www.agingwithdignity.org/five-wishes. php*
- American Bar Association: *www.abanet.org/publiced/practical/ directive_whatis.html*

- Caring Connections from the National Hospice and Palliative Care Organization: *caringinfo.org/i4a/pages/index.cfm?pageid=3289*
- US Living Wills Registry: *liv-will1.uslivingwillregistry.com/forms.html*
- The Departments of Health in individual states

Guardianship and Conservatorship

Guardianships and conservatorships are legal relationships created by the court whereby a person or professional organization is appointed to protect people who cannot handle their own financial or personal affairs. Definitions vary from state to state. Most generally, a **guardian** is appointed for the purpose of managing the personal affairs of a person who has become incapacitated (called a ward), including making personal decisions and meeting needs for medical care, nutrition, clothing, shelter, or safety. A **conservator** is appointed for a person (called a protected person) for the purpose of managing finances, assets, and income when it has been shown that the person has impaired ability and/or judgment. If a person needs both a guardian and a conservator, one person may be appointed by the court to fill both of those roles.

A Guardianship or Conservatorship Is Required When No Plan Is in Place

A guardianship or conservatorship is necessary when a person becomes unable to handle finances or live safely without help and no previous arrangements have been made. The decision to obtain a guardianship or conservatorship should not be made lightly because it takes away the person's most basic right: to make decisions about his or her own health and welfare. The court will appoint a guardian or conservator who will handle all of the person's affairs, including perhaps where he or she will live. The court will appoint a guardian or conservator only if a less restrictive alternative is not available. It is likely that neither a guardianship nor conservatorship will be necessary if a healthcare directive and a power of attorney have been put into place.

Establishment of a Guardianship or Conservatorship

While practices may vary state by state, generally a guardianship or conservatorship is established by filing a petition with the probate court in the county where the person resides. Anyone can ask the court to appoint a guardian or conservator for a person who needs help. The potential ward or protected person must be given advance notice of the hearing and has the right to be represented by an attorney at any court proceeding, even if he or she cannot pay for the attorney. In this case, the court will order the county to pay these costs. The person requesting a guardianship or conservatorship must prove through clear and convincing evidence that such an order is necessary. This could be difficult if the proposed ward or protected person does not want a guardianship or conservatorship established.

Your Will

A **will** is a set of written instructions about how to dispose of your assets upon death. Assets are either described as probate assets or nonprobate assets. Probate assets are those assets whose ownership a court must rule on following the owner's death. Nonprobate assets are assets that will automatically transfer to another person at death such as those with joint tenancy or beneficiary designations or assets that have been placed in a trust. Probate court is the court charged with determining ownership either by administering a legal will or by state law when no legal will exists.

Not Everyone Needs a Will—But It Is a Good Idea

If property is held in such a way that it will pass through beneficiary designations or joint ownership, then a will is not technically necessary. However, a will is necessary if a person wants personal property, such as jewelry, paintings, and family heirlooms, distributed in a certain way. Tax or private family matters may exist that make it wise to use a will and probate court to administer an estate. Finally, even if there seems to be no reason for a will, having one is the best way to ensure that an individual's wishes will be followed.

GLOSSARY

antigen: a substance that provokes an immune response.

ataxia: a significant loss of muscle coordination. It can occur in the limbs, the trunk, or with walking.

autoimmune disease: when the body's immune system is mistakenly attacking and damaging healthy tissues.

autonomic nervous system: the "control system" that governs the body's reflexive, automatic functions—things that happen without our conscious thought, such as heart rate, digestion, respiration rate, salivation, and perspiration.

axons: Wire-like extensions of the cells that send messages from one part of the brain to another.

blood-brain barrier: highly selective, semi-permeable blood vessels that form a barrier between the circulating blood and the brain, allowing some necessary cells into the brain, but restricting other cells that could be harmful.

central nervous system (CNS): composed of the brain and spinal cord and optic nerve, the CNS coordinates the activity of all parts of the body.

cerebrospinal fluid (CSF): a clear, watery fluid that is continuously produced and absorbed and that flows in the ventricles within the brain and around the surface of the brain and spinal cord.

chromosome: DNA containing structures in cells.

clinically isolated syndrome: when someone has a first neurologic attack that is consistent with central nervous system inflammation.

cranial nerves: twelve pairs of nerves that originate in the brain or brainstem that control specific sensory and motor functions, particularly those involving the eyes, ears, nose, mouth, throat, face and neck.

disease-modifying therapies: those drugs that modify the underlying mechanism of the disease itself, rather than just temporarily alleviating symptoms.

dysesthesia: unpleasant, abnormal sense of touch.

dysmetria: the undershooting and overshooting of the intended movement or target.

epidemiologic studies: studies of how diseases behave in different populations and different locations.

evoked potential studies: tests of the nerve pathways from the vision, hearing, or sensation centers to the brain.

evoked potentials: also called "evoked responses," are recordings of the nerves' response to various stimuli.

executive function: a set of mental processes that helps connect past experience with present action; important for decision making, planning and organizing.

foot drop: gait abnormality characterized by limited or no ability to lift the foot.

gait: a person's manner of walking.

gray matter: one of two primary components of the central nervous system, consisting largely of neuronal cell bodies.

immune system: a system of biological structures and processes that protects against disease by attacking foreign "intruders," such as viruses, bacteria, parasites, and cancer cells.

inflammation: a carefully orchestrated response of the immune system to threats such as injury, irritation or infection.

irrevocable trust: a separate taxable entity, requiring its own tax identification number; cannot be changed or terminated after it has
been established.

lassitude: an overwhelming sense of tiredness that materializes out
of the blue. It is not necessarily associated with exertion or heat
exposure, but in some instances it can be exacerbated by factors
such as heat, stress, sleep disruption, or medications.

living trust: the type of trust used to manage assets during a time of
incapacity.

lumbar puncture: the procedure of taking fluid from the space around
the spinal cord in the lower back through a hollow needle, usually
done for diagnostic purposes.

magnetic resonance imaging (MRI): a technique that uses a magnetic
field and radio waves to create detailed images of the organs and
tissues within the body.

major histocompatibility complex (MHC): regions on chromosomes
that control the development and function of many immune
components.

multiple sclerosis: often referred to as MS, multiple sclerosis is a
chronic disease that affects the body's central nervous system, or
brain and spinal cord, and commonly produces symptoms that can
include fatigue, numbness, weakness, vision change, and loss of
balance—among others.

muscle tone: how loose or stiff the muscles are.

myelin: a fatty substance, wrapped around most nerves, that both protects the nerve fibers and accelerates nerve-impulse transmission.

nerve cells: the core components of the nervous system, which process
and transmit information to and from the brain and spinal cord
based on electrical and chemical signaling.

nerve fiber fatigue: with heat exposure or exertion, someone with MS
may experience a temporary worsening of a neurologic symptom.

nerve impulses: waves of chemical and electrical excitement that travel
along nerve fibers in response to a stimulus.

neurologist: a medical specialist in the nervous system and the disorders affecting it.

neuropsychologist: a physiologist who specializes in understanding the relationship between the physical brain and behavior.

occipital neuralgia: causes pain in the distribution of the occipital nerve.

oligodendrocytes: the myelin-forming cells in the central nervous system.

optic nerve: the nerve (one for each eye) that transmits visual information from the retina to the brain.

optic neuritis: inflammation of the optic nerve causing vision impairment in one eye.

paresthesia: an abnormal sensation, typically tingling or pricking.

peripheral nervous system (PNS): extends throughout the body, and is responsible for connecting the central nervous system to the limbs and organs.

plaques: scar tissues.

periodic plateaus: periods when the disease is stable.

power of attorney: a written document in which you (as the "principal") appoint another person (the "attorney-in-fact") to handle your property or finances.

primary MS fatigue: the sense of feeling tired, either physically, cognitively or both that results directly from the MS disease process.

primary-progressive MS: a course marked by a slow decline in neurologic function from the start, with no sharply identifiable relapses or remissions.

proprioception: awareness of the position of one's body.

pseudo-exacerbations: a person experiences a new or worsened neurologic symptom as a result of overexertion, becoming overheated, or an infection (such as a cold or a bladder infection); the symptoms are real, but the underlying cause is something besides MS.

relapsing-remitting: occurs when an individual develops neurologic symptoms that last a minimum of 24 hours and cannot be explained by any other cause, such as an infection. The symptoms remain for a period of weeks to months and then completely or partially resolve.

residual symptoms: the remaining symptoms, when recovery is less than 100%.

restless legs syndrome: unpleasant tickling or twitching sensation in the leg muscles when sitting or lying down, which is relieved only by moving the legs.

revocable trust: normally used for property management purposes; cannot be changed or terminated after it has been established. It is a separate taxable entity, requiring its own tax identification number.

secondary MS fatigue: the sense of feeling tired that is provoked by a non-MS source such as another illness, depression, stress, medication side effects, poor sleep, or over exertion.

secondary-progressive MS: the disease worsens rather steadily and may or may not include periodic plateaus occasional relapses, and minor remissions.

sensory ataxia: unsteady walking, standing or other movements due to disruption in the spinal cord or brain that interferes with the nerves carrying information about the position of the body and/or limbs.

somatosensory nervous system: The receptors and processors that allow our senses to react to stimuli and comprehend things such as touch, temperature, body position, and pain.

spasm: a sudden tightening of muscles in an arm or leg.

spasticity: a chronic state of excessive muscle tone (too much tension in the muscles).

stem cell: a cell that is capable of developing into another type of cell.

testamentary trust: a trust created by the terms of the grantor's will.

tremors: involuntary rhythmic movements of a given body part, usually an arm or leg.

trigeminal neuralgia: facial pain, sometimes quite intense, that travels along one of the three branches of the trigeminal nerve, which supplies sensation to the face.

white matter: the other primary component of the central nervous system, consisting largely of axons sheathed in a protective coating of myelin, an insulating material.

About the American Academy of Neurology

The American Academy of Neurology, an association of more than 28,000 neurologists and neuroscience professionals, is dedicated to promoting the highest quality patient-centered neurologic care. A neurologist is a doctor with specialized training in diagnosing, treating, and managing disorders of the brain and nervous system such as Alzheimer's disease, stroke, migraine, multiple sclerosis, concussion, Parkinson's disease, and epilepsy.

For more information about the American Academy of Neurology, visit *AAN.com*.

To sign up for a free subscription to *Neurology Now*, the Academy's magazine for patients and caregivers, visit *NeurologyNow.com*.

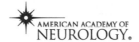

About the American Brain Foundation

The American Brain Foundation, the foundation of the American Academy of Neurology, supports crucial research and education to discover causes, improved treatments, and cures for the brain and other nervous system diseases. One in six people is affected by brain diseases such as Alzheimer's disease, traumatic brain injury, stroke, Parkinson's disease, multiple sclerosis, autism, and epilepsy.

For more information about the American Brain Foundation and how you can support research, visit *AmericanBrainFoundation.org*.

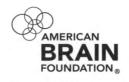

175

INDEX

Page numbers followed by *f* or *t* indicate figures or tables, respectively. Numbers in *italics* indicate boxed text.